HEALING
After Birth

Navigating Your Emotions After A Difficult Childbirth

JENNIFER SUMMERFELDT, MACP

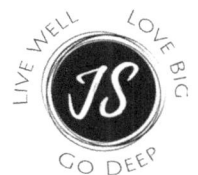

JS Coaching
EDMONTON, ALBERTA

Copyright © 2018 by Jennifer Summerfeldt.

All rights reserved. No part of this publication may be reproduced, distributed or transmitted in any form or by any means, including photocopying, recording, or other electronic or mechanical methods, without the prior written permission of the publisher, except in the case of brief quotations embodied in critical reviews and certain other noncommercial uses permitted by copyright law. For permission requests, write to the publisher, addressed "Attention: Permissions Coordinator," at the address below.

Jennifer Summerfeldt/JS Coaching

Edmonton/Alberta/Canada

www.jennifersummerfeldt.com

Layout and Typography by Greg deJong

Ordering Information:

Quantity sales. Special discounts are available on quantity purchases by corporations, associations, and others. For details, contact the "Special Sales Department" at the address above.

Healing After Birth/ Jennifer Summerfeldt. —1st ed.

ISBN 978-1-9994972-0-0

Contents

Foreword	i
Preface	iii
Introduction	v
SELF-ASSESSMENT	
Was Your Birth Traumatic?	xiii
REFLECTIVE EXERCISE	
Know Your 'Why'	xvii
CHAPTER 1	
My Birth Story	
Told Without Shame	1
CHAPTER 2	
Setting the Stage for Healing	15
REFLECTIVE EXERCISE	
On Safety & Grounding	21
CHAPTER 3	
Understanding Shame	23
REFLECTIVE EXERCISE	
On Shame	33
THERAPEUTIC ACTIVITY	
Narrative Exercise	35
CHAPTER 4	
Understanding Trauma	37
REFLECTIVE EXERCISE	
On Trauma	43
THERAPEUTIC ACTIVITY	
Visualization Exercise	45

CHAPTER 5	
How Birth Can Involve Trauma	47
REFLECTIVE EXERCISE	
On Childbirth Trauma	53
Deeper Reading	55
CHAPTER 6	
Making Sense of Your Grief	63
REFLECTIVE EXERCISE	
On Grief	73
CHAPTER 7	
Letting Go of Blame and Anger	75
REFLECTIVE EXERCISE	
On Anger and Blame	81
THERAPEUTIC ACTIVITY	
Narrative Exercise	84
CHAPTER 8	
Learning to Trust	
Your Body Again	91
REFLECTIVE EXERCISE	
On Anger and Blame	101
THERAPEUTIC ACTIVITY	
Narrative Exercise	104
CHAPTER 9	
Learning to	
See Things Differently	105
REFLECTIVE EXERCISE	
Building Compassion	117
REFLECTIVE EXERCISE	
Revisiting Your Why	119

CHAPTER 10
    Exploring Meaning
    in Motherhood   121
REFLECTIVE EXERCISE
    On the Postpartum   127
On Mindfulness and Motherhood   131
THERAPEUTIC ACTIVITY
    Embracing Yourself
    as a Loving Mother   137
NARRATIVE EXERCISE   139

CHAPTER 11
    Reclaiming Your Birth Story   141
On Vulnerability   142
REFLECTIVE EXERCISE
    Your Birth Story   149
THERAPEUTIC ACTIVITY
    Narrative Exercise   151
"One Day I Will Rage"   157

References   159

This guidebook is dedicated to all of the mothers who have courageously stepped forward and said yes to their healing. To the teachers and healers who have influenced my work along the way: Marea Butler, Whapio Diane Bartlett, Jane Simington, Bonnie Badenoch, and Amanda Slugoski. To my children, whom without, I would not have my passion. To my dearest sister and friend who has held me through it all. To my parents for continuing to believe in me despite my radical viewpoints. And finally, to my loving soul companion. Without his unwavering belief in me, I am not sure I would have had the strength, stamina, and courage to heal.

Sometimes you just have to remind yourself that there is purpose in the chaos. Always breathe deeper into it. Trust that eventually, after all the debris has settled, there is a tender core awaiting your return.

Foreword

Healing after Birth is a book full of wisdom, practical help, and generous, courageous truth telling. It addresses our need as a world to heal trauma experienced during birth. I am deeply grateful Jennifer wrote this book. This book can help you heal.

Our original prenatal, birth and newborn experiences set the template for all our relationship patterns with: ourselves, our bodies, each other, the earth, and spirit as we know it.

Ample research over the recent decades has revealed the profound lifelong impact left by violence, trauma, disrespect and lack of genuine caring during the prenatal, birth, and newborn stages of life. As Dr. Michael Lu, the author of the Life Course Model, points out, without healing treatment or positive mitigating circumstances, early traumatic experiences lead to a lifelong low tolerance for stress, a predisposition for illness, and a strong tendency to neglect and/or abuse self and others.

Perinatal Trauma can be healed. Go through the chapters and exercises in this book. As Jennifer points out in this book, when we resolve perinatal trauma, we receive gifts of high value. We can experience feeling safe and calm in our bodies again rather than feeling frozen or in a state of hyperarousal. We can experience an ease and openness with our love for our babies and close ones rather than feeling guilt, shame, rage and low self-esteem. We reconnect with ourselves, our babies, our relationships.

This book honors the need for women, partners and perinatal professionals who have had traumatic or difficult experiences to be seen and recognized. It gives an effective path for resolution of these experiences. It includes self-respect, compassion and grounding, for one's experience throughout the healing path. That is why it is effective. Weaving feelings of safety to open to what needs to be healed and then returning to feeling safe again allows healing.

As a Perinatal EMDR Certified Psychotherapist over the last several decades, I have worked with hundreds of mothers, partners and perinatal professionals, individually and in groups and have seen perinatal trauma resolved. I have also developed an effective model for treating Perinatal Trauma individually and in groups.

I recommend this book to mothers and perinatal professionals. This book offers in detail, in a user-friendly way, the same precepts I base my effective and successful perinatal healing trauma model on.

Jennifer's book also clarifies how many of our current obstetric medical model care systems contribute unintentionally to some women's experience of trauma. Understanding this helps demystify tremendous guilt and confusion for people who experienced birth trauma in these systems and were never validated.

When women who experienced and perceived themselves as having birth trauma are sent home without validation, women can feel "crazy" for experiencing trauma symptoms, but not knowing why. In an ideal situation, from the understandings in Jennifer's book, it would be helpful and supportive if women were told:

"You had an experience that you might have perceived as traumatic, life threatening, being out of control. Here are some of the symptoms you might experience. Here are some of the practices that will help you. Here are resources that can help you as well. We are here to help."

Jennifer explains why this occurs and this is validating and healing in itself. This impressive book is very comprehensive. It combines science with compassion and effective interventions and reveals clearly what has been mystified and unclear for a long time.

In reading **Healing after Birth**, I received further personal healing. In the birth of my son, I did not experience trauma birthing him. The actual birth, however, as happens for many people, stimulated my limbic memory of my own traumatic birth into our world. As soon as the postpartum period began, I began to experience the painful trigger symptoms of trauma: hyperarousal, disassociation, depression and more. I did not understand then what I know now and what this book explains so well about trauma. I felt ashamed to be feeling the way I did and felt I was a bad mother. Jennifer's compassion and clarity about the roots of mother shame and her exercises to cut through it supported me to make an appointment with a perinatal psychotherapist. This therapy allowed me to heal a significant traumatic experience I had as a newborn. This has positively affected my current relationship with my adult son. For the first time, I didn't have constant tension while experiencing our relationship, and his beauty and care. What a Gift! It is never too late to heal. Thank-you Jennifer!!!

Gena McCarthy, RN, MFT — www.BirthSpiritualityandHealing.com

PREFACE

Your body did not fail you.
You did nothing wrong.
You are not alone.

Dear Mother,

Millions of mothers around the world suffer in silence after a difficult birthing experience. Why? In some cases, it's because they're led to believe that their experience was normal and that they need to "just get over it". In other cases, it's because they're told to focus on being happy that they have a new baby. But secretly, many of these mothers wonder: "What is wrong with me? Why can't I get over what happened? Why don't I feel happy? Am I not cut out to be a mother?"

This guidebook is dedicated to every mother who endured unexpected overwhelming challenges and difficulties during her labour and delivery and was sent home without any acknowledgment of what had just taken place. It's for every mother who was left alone with grief and confusion yet expected to transition easily and quickly into her role as a new mother.

This guidebook is for mothers of all walks of life and from all generations—the mothers who years ago were strapped to their beds, drugged, told to be quiet, to the mothers who will hopefully one day give birth in an environment that respects the sacredness of women's bodies and motherhood.

Finally, this guidebook is for humanity, encouraging us all to recognize that a healthy society is one that honours the birthing experience and places mothers at the apex of that experience.

Introduction

Vision, Motivation and Goals of this Guidebook

Birth is a transformative process that can result in both profound pain and profound bliss. When a mother is unwell, the family is unwell, and the community is unwell. Mothers need to be at the centre – not at the edge – of our society.

I created the **Healing After Birth** program in response to the World Health Organization's statement in 2015 that encouraged health professionals to address the rising rates of childbirth trauma[1]. Childbirth trauma has both immediate and long-term mental health implications for the entire family system.

However, the seeds of the **Healing After Birth** program were planted long before that. Since 1999, I have been immersed in the childbirth continuum and worn many hats: advocate, researcher, educator, doula, author and direct-entry midwifery student and apprentice. These experiences led me to combine experiential and learned knowledge to create a comprehensive group program that is both trauma-informed and healing.

The overarching goal of the **Healing After Birth** program is to offer a trauma-informed perspective that assists in repairing fragile and fractured attachment bonds between mothers and their family units due to childbirth trauma.

This guidebook was developed out of the **Healing After Birth** program. It can be used in conjunction with the program or as a standalone tool. The intention of this guidebook is to enhance family wellbeing and help mothers engage in their new role with meaning and a sense of emotional and mental wellness.

Many of today's mothers find it difficult to talk about their experiences openly and honestly. More often than not, they experience loneliness and isolation, even when they attend play groups. They struggle to have real conversations with other moms due to (perceived?) competition about birth and childrearing. This has been expressed to me over and over in a survey I conducted and throughout my clinical practice.

Because of these struggles, many mothers place an expectation on their primary partner to meet their emotional needs and relieve them from the burdens of daily life. This adds stress to an already stressful environment and their relationships can start to weaken or fracture.

---

[1] WHO, "The Prevention and Elimination of Disrespect and Abuse During Facility-Based Childbirth," 2015. http://apps.who.int/iris/bitstream/10665/134588/1/WHO_RHR_14.23_eng.pdf

The stress of the postpartum period is real. When adding the emotional weight of having experienced a traumatic or difficult childbirth and the worries of "catching" a mood disorder, everything becomes more challenging. Thus, many of today's mothers experience their early encounters with motherhood as stressful and isolating. The amount of information available at our fingertips only increases concerns. Mothers can easily become frozen and afraid to move in any direction for fear of "doing it wrong" or "being a bad mother".

And, there are still far too many mothers who are in survival mode due to historical trauma, violence, oppression, marginalization, and discrimination due to race, creed, or religion. And for the mothers who are struggling to stay alive within a dominant world view that devalues their humanity, need alone their motherhood, my body rages and walks alongside you as an ally. I see you and honour you, and I can only imagine the huge barriers you face to move beyond survival towards a thriving life. You are not alone, nor do you need to heal alone. My hope is that the collective work of all mothers, who *can* engage in their healing, will do their work, so we can hold hope together that you too shall step out of terror, and into a collective community of dignity, love and authentic honouring.

This guidebook will help mothers who are struggling to make sense of their birthing experience (and their new role as a mother) *shift out* of a state of hurt, pain, isolation, panic, fear, paralysis and insecurity. It will help them process the stored emotional and mental material held within their bodies and psyche. It will inspire them to trust that they can heal and move forward as experts of their babies and their process. And, it will help them access resources if they get stuck.

Most importantly, this guidebook will help mothers see that they are *enough*. Peace.

A Bit About Me

My passion for helping mothers find emotional wellness emerged in 1999 when I was pregnant with my first child. I would have never anticipated that my first pregnancy would have resulted in a lifelong passion to serve women during their childbearing years. After reading too many books to count, there are some fundamental themes that have motivated my passion:

- ★ How we experience birth is a human rights issue and women's rights issue.
- ★ Childbirth is an extension of the mother's sexual health.
- ★ Instinctive childbirth is not generally supported by the mainstream medical establishment.
- ★ Women are violated frequently throughout labour and birth, often without acknowledgment.
- ★ Mothers are often isolated and overwhelmed in the postpartum period.
- ★ Motherhood is not at the centre of our society but rather at the edge. In other words, we do not value the act of mothering as an important contribution to a healthy society.
- ★ Obstetrical violence is real, and has been real, since it entered into the birthing milieu at the turn of the 20th century.
- ★ Newborns are emotional, responsive, sentient beings.
- ★ Postpartum mood disorders are at the forefront of today's childbirth conversations.
- ★ Our deepest wounds are attachment wounds, which can begin in utero.
- ★ All of these themes have given rise to a fire inside of me. I feel that there are deep injustices (and at times overt violence) in the way that most women experience childbirth. And it's been like that for generations.

I remember asking both of my grandmothers years ago about their childbirth experiences. I was horrified to learn that they both endured traumatic births. My maternal grandmother was 17 years old and utterly confused and terrified throughout her labour because she didn't understand how her baby was going to come out. She was so disconnected from her body and the process that the medical staff responded by strapping her to the bed and telling her to stop whining. Eventually, amidst her terror and confusion, my mother was born. My grandmother described it as horrifying.

My adopted paternal grandmother experienced something similar; however, she gave birth during the era of twilight sleep. She told me that she was forced to take sleeping medication, passed out, and woke up with a baby by her side. The nurses told her that although she wouldn't remember anything about the birth, she had acted like a wild animal and needed to be strapped to the bed.

Stories like these fuels the fire within me. It's this fire that has brought me to the place I am at today. It's the same fire that drives me to want to serve mothers who have experienced unexpected, difficult or traumatic births and who are struggling in the postpartum period.

I created the ***Healing After Birth*** program and this guidebook out of an accumulation of experiences over my lifetime. This includes my years spent as a performance psychology graduate student, a student of neurobiology and trauma theory (before trauma-informed care entered the mainstream conversation), and a graduate student in counselling psychology. I am fortunate to have had the privilege to access these teachings and further my education. **I believe those who have privilege have a responsibility to use their privilege wisely.**

I acknowledge that I am a white woman, born into a middle-class family with two working parents. Although I faced childhood traumas, I have had access to resources along the way that served to support me in my healing journey. I was gifted with a natural athletic talent, which gave me an outlet to express myself and led me to a scholarship in university. My path throughout university was long and winding; however, I have over 9 years of traditional academic studies, including studies in two graduate programs with a master's in counselling psychology.

I recognize that attending a university is a privilege. Playing high level sports is also a privilege. Being raised within a family with financial resources is a privilege. Having an extended family that loved me is a privilege. Accessing midwifery care and paying for it, even when I was low income, is a privilege. And being white, in North America, is a privilege. **Therefore, I acknowledge that I write from a place of privilege.** My hope is that I can share from this place and offer insight and support to those who have not had the same privileges.

I also honour and note that the amount of privilege one holds has an impact on their birthing experience. Those who have been marginalized or whom hold unresolved historical and intergenerational trauma face more barriers within the milieu of childbirth.

To people who are transgender, who struggle to relate to the notion of 'motherhood', or who do not align with the binary gender words *woman* or *she*, I acknowledge you and the additional stressors you experience throughout the childbearing times. I also acknowledge that the complexity of gender politics, reproductive politics, and that patriarchy runs rampant throughout the childbearing atmosphere. Although I do not speak specifically in this guidebook about the additional complexities that transgender, gender queer or gender non-conforming people may experience, I do recognize that this exists, requires attention and deserves to be included in the conversations at large.

That said, throughout this guidebook I use the words *motherhood*, *woman*, and *she* to speak to the audience at large. I also unpack the notion of motherhood as a verb, rather than a gender specific term. I hold a strong desire to inspire people who have given birth to claim the role and the word: Mother.

Finally, I am blessed to say that this work is incredibly meaningful. I am incredibly grateful to witness mothers around the world heal and embrace motherhood with confidence, meaning and love.

What to Expect

Throughout this guidebook you will be led through a healing journey that intends to foster integration and coherence within the following areas: mind, brain, heart, body, and family. It will help you make sense of your childbirth experience and postpartum struggles.

Each reflective exercise encourages you to actively engage in your healing. The key word is: *engage*. Without active engagement, nothing will change. The deeper your commitment and readiness for the journey that lies ahead, the greater your results will be. I invite you to hold the intention that healing is possible. Each chapter in this guidebook has a teaching component plus reflective activities and the option to access further therapeutic exercises through my membership site.

It is recommended that you not rush the process. Healing cannot be rushed. You may feel the urge to go through the activities quickly in hopes that the sooner you 'get it done' the quicker you will feel better. But I am inviting you to consider healing as a process rather than a commodity.

Healing is not something that can be consumed or bought. We are bombarded with information these days, more than ever. I don't know about you, but my brain is full. I cannot consume more information or programs.

This program is aligned in a way that encourages you to have a lived experience of the material and engage in the 'felt' experience, rather than just a 'thought' experience.

> **Bottom line: We do not heal from thinking alone.**
> We cannot 'think' our way out of our pain.
> We need to feel our way through the challenges.
> We need to feel our way through the pain.

I encourage you to invest in one chapter per week. Slower is better for integration. Return to the previous section if you find you are challenged to move forward. Notice and observe in between lessons. Pay attention to small shifts in your body, mind, heart and relationships. And, finally, trust the innate intelligence within you that seeks wholeness and integration. We heal from the inside out, not the outside in. You are the expert of your process and the answers lie within the seat of your heart.

Guidebook Flow

- ★ Begin with your Why
- ★ Establish safety and grounding to go deep into your healing
- ★ Become informed about healing and trauma recovery
- ★ Go down and under to access unprocessed memories, feelings and felt sensations
- ★ Process, reprocess, reorganize and reprogram
- ★ Reconnect to life and love
- ★ Reclaim yourself as a mother
- ★ Create meaning and find purpose

Guiding Assumptions

The following perspectives support the foundational viewpoints of this guidebook:

1. We are shaped by our environment as early as in utero.
2. Our early childhood experiences give rise to our programs—how we think, feel, and behave.
3. How we make sense of early childhood experiences, especially adversities, makes up the foundation of our limiting core beliefs.
4. We experience our present reality through the lens of our past, until we become conscious of it.
5. Traumatic material gets stored and stuck in our biological system and needs to be discharged.
6. The brain seeks to make sense of everything.
7. We are always telling ourselves something about the presenting situation.
8. We are always telling ourselves something about 'oneself' in relation to our present situation.
9. Traumatic experiences, if left unresolved, remain on repeat—dumping stress chemicals into our system, resulting in illness (including mental illness) and dysregulation.

10. Grief, when felt with presence, opens the heart.
11. Holding the felt experiences (sensations within the body) with presence supports integration.
12. Our mind cannot differentiate between inner world vs outer world—both are real.
13. Our core wounds give rise to profound wisdom when integrated.
14. There is a way through the emotional pain of our past and it is within us to find the way.
15. You do not need to be defined by your past experiences.
16. You are awareness experiencing your biology and life.
17. Perception (how we make sense out of) of environmental information (experiences) signals the expression of a gene.
18. There is a field that contains information and energy, and we are interconnected to this field and in communion with it at all times. Some people call this field *consciousness*.

Program Outcomes

As you work through this guidebook, you can expect:
- ★ To build your capacity to identify and express emotions related to your childbirth experience.
- ★ To decrease postpartum symptoms of anxiety and/or depression as a result of your unresolved childbirth trauma.
- ★ To grieve what was lost during your birth experience.
- ★ To learn how to regulate your nervous system.
- ★ To learn how to be present with what is arising and know what to do with that information.
- ★ To shift cognitive perspectives about your birth experience and integrate a new narrative that feels whole and complete.
- ★ To increase your knowledge about healthy, secure attachments and to practice this with your baby.
- ★ To become trauma informed and understand that you did nothing wrong.
- ★ To increase self-awareness and engage more regularly with a mindfulness practice while mothering.
- ★ To decrease fears associated with childbirth.
- ★ To know you are not alone.

Getting Started

To get started, make sure you have a calm and secure space to engage with the process that follows. Choose a buddy—a friend, partner, parent, colleague, therapist, or other trusted person that you can call on if you need additional support to process what is coming to the surface. Finally, *believe* that healing is possible—that you can feel better and different about your childbirth experience.

You are responsible for your healing journey. Only you can discover the healing you crave. Guides can support, help, provide insight, gently challenge and hold space for your growth and healing. However, the magic lies within you. There is an intelligence within that wants to guide you towards healing and wholeness.

Before you begin this healing journey, it is important that you set up space in your home and within your calendar. Imagine that this program is akin to meeting weekly with a local support group. This way you will flow into the exercises at a healing pace.

One of the challenges with any program, especially those that are therapeutic in nature, is that people can lack commitment to the process. I am not sitting with you in person, therefore it is easy to half engage in the activities. However, part of healing is realizing that you are in charge of the process.

> To deepen your healing experience, you are invited to apply to the **Healing After Birth Program** in which you will receive 6 one-on-one sessions PLUS weekly videos, audios, guided meditations, and therapeutic activities. If you are not ready to engage with this level of therapeutic support, you can sign up for a BONUS audio to support inner resourcing and connecting to your calm place. Both intended to help you feel supported and held as you dive into healing your birth experience. Head on over to www.jennifersummerfeldt.com and click on 'FREE Audio' link to access the audio files.

SELF-ASSESSMENT

Was Your Birth Traumatic?

As we explore the concept of birth trauma, you may or may not identify with the term. Either way is okay. However, take a moment to answer *yes, no, I don't know,* to the following questions:

* Did you experience an overwhelming amount of pain at any point during your labour?
* Did you experience any sense of floating, disconnecting, or disembodying, at any point?
* Did you see yourself outside of your body, as if you were looking down on yourself?
* Did you interpret at any point that you or your baby were in harm's way?
* Did you feel at any point utter overwhelm or an absolute lack of control?
* Did you wish you could have fought or run out of the room, but you were trapped and couldn't?
* Did you feel any sensation of physiological panic or terror?
* Did you feel any numbness or tingling throughout your body?
* Did you wish you could have screamed or said something but couldn't because you felt frozen or too afraid to speak up?
* Did you experience any flashbacks in which you were reminded of past traumatic experiences?
* At any point during your labour did you perceive that you were violated, attacked or forced to do something against your will?
* Did you feel, or do you now feel, a sense of disconnection from yourself and/or your baby or partner—like they were strangers?
* Do you avoid thinking about your childbirth experience?
* Did you try to speak up during labour only to have your needs ignored, resulting in a feeling of disempowerment?

If you answered *yes* to any of the above statements, chances are you experienced giving birth as an extremely stressful event—maybe even traumatic. That said, answering *yes* without taking into consideration your current perception of the event is only part of the equation. Two people can experience a similar event, yet each can interpret, and therefore store, the information of the event differently.

Important questions to consider since you gave birth:
* When you think about the event, are you flooded with negative emotions, sensations, or thoughts?
* Do you avoid thinking about your past birth experience?
* Are you harbouring unresolved emotions?
* Are you stuck in blame or shame?
* Do you fear giving birth again?
* Are you glad it's over with and do you never want to revisit that experience?
* Are you having nightmares and/or difficulty sleeping and finding calm?
* Are you struggling with symptoms of depression and/or anxiety?
* Are you hypervigilant, or do you get the sense that you are always on guard?
* Are you feeling numb, distant, and disconnected from yourself and others?
* Does it seem like life is happening around you, but you're not a part of it?
* Are you struggling to communicate your thoughts effectively?
* When you think back to your birth, does it feel like a blur, as if pieces are missing?
* Does it feel like it just happened yesterday, even if it has been weeks, months, or years?
* Does the event haunt you throughout the day or night?
* Does it feel like the birth happened to someone else and not you?
* Do you get sudden flashes in your mind throughout the day or night?

Answering *yes* to any of these questions can indicate that the stressful material—memories, sensations, emotions, and thoughts—is likely trapped within your nervous system, mind and heart. You are likely stuck in a stress response due to unresolved emotions, thoughts, sensations, and memories pertaining to your birth. Of course, for a professional diagnosis it is recommended that you visit your medical professional.

What do your answers to the questions above say about your current situation? They tell you that your system needs your kind attention to help it return to a state of health and wellness. The good news is this can be done. You do not have to remain in overdrive and distress for the remainder of your postpartum time or journey into motherhood. To heal, we have to get our mental health to a place where our system is in a state of coherence[2]. But more on that later.

---

2   Daniel Siegel, *"The Mindful Brain: The Neurobiology of Wellbeing"* (2001), doi:978-1-60407-227-3; Daniel J Siegel, *Mindsight: The New Science of Personal Transformation* (New York: Random House Publishing Group, 2010).

The final big questions to consider, when assessing if your birth was traumatic:
- ★ As you think about your past experience of giving birth, how do you feel?
- ★ When you think about and tell your birth story, how would you like to feel?
- ★ What is preventing you from feeling and thinking differently about your birth story?
- ★ Who or what is in charge of making those changes?
- ★ Do you desire to feel better?
- ★ Are you willing to invest in your health?

If there is still trauma stuck in your system, it is imperative that you receive the necessary support to help you discharge the stressful information. This guidebook alone cannot help you release the stress from your body, but it can act as a companion by helping you move through any stuck emotions and foster a new birth story.

Working with a professional who is trauma-informed—a psychologist, counselor, body therapist, spiritual/shamanic practitioner, or energy therapist—is an essential component towards restoring your nervous system back to health.

I call this the "getting my brain back online" stage of healing. Yet, your healing will not feel complete until you have integrated all the aspects of your birth experience. **This includes changing the way you tell your story and feel about the event.** Trust me, the story does change. When we begin to heal, we have a wider gaze in which we can hold many different aspects of the experience at once. We are no longer stuck in only the negative memories, but rather, the story becomes fluid and moving. In fact, the birth story is always moving. It is alive.

Let's recap:
a. You asked yourself hard questions;
b. You evaluated how stressful the event was;
c. You considered if your body, mind and heart is still hanging on to the stressful material; and
d. You asked yourself an important question about how you want to think and feel about your birth.

Great. I am so glad you are diving into this journey. Let's continue!

REFLECTIVE EXERCISE
KNOW YOUR 'WHY'

Why did you choose this guidebook?

What do you hope to experience?

Why have you decided to invest in your healing?

What feels unfinished in regard to your birth?

What thoughts, images and feelings still swirl around and keep you up at night?

What has been holding you back from healing?

CHAPTER 1

MY BIRTH STORY
told without shame

Now that you've reflected on your Why, I want to interject with a personal story. I've included the story of my birth here for a few reasons:

> Stories are powerful ways to communicate a point.
> Stories connect and normalize.
> Stories help us discover meaning.
> Stories inform us and others where we might be stuck.
> Stories validate knowledge.
> Stories are healing.

I was indecisive about including this story as part of this guidebook, until my editor highlighted the power within the story. In fact, I noticed that I was considering withholding this story for the same reasons that many of the mothers I work with withhold sharing the truth about their birthing experiences—a belief that it is not valid, does not belong, or is not 'bad' enough to be recounted.

Deeper yet, there is and was a fear that the sharing of the birth story will not be validated; that I/we will be judged. So, we tell parts of it and we edit the content of our own birth story to fit the group narrative of the time. We desperately want to belong and so we make our stories fit by removing or adding pieces to dilute the experience.

What this tells me is that even amongst groups of close mothers we are afraid to be authentic and vulnerable with how we really feel about our experience of giving birth. And yet, the antidote lies within the courage to be vulnerable.

The following is a recount of the raw, honest, reflection of the fullness of my birth experiences that encompasses both absolute awe and power, as well as utter chaos and terror.

In reflecting upon this notion that both awe and terror were present within my birth experience, I am *now* not surprised (albeit I was horrified at the time). This proves to me how our stories change as we mend together the broken pieces and make sense of it all. For example: I understand that we live in a 3D reality in which duality exists. Science tells us that the whole contains both light and dark, in union and relation to one another. One cannot exist without the other. From this perspective, I can hold that both the extremes of great joy *and* pain coincided within my birth experience.

On that note, I will begin to unravel my birth story.
How did I come to know shame intimately as a mother? Was it because I was carrying a secret about my birth for the past 12 years? Here I am, offering counselling and facilitating a program I created called **Healing After Birth**, and yet I believed that I didn't have a traumatic or difficult birth. My three deliveries were all at home and empowering, so I thought.

I can reflect upon the voices of the mothers who have said to me: "My birth was great, nothing was wrong with it, I am okay with what happened during my birth experience. I am not struggling because of the birth, it is something else."

Yet, when we explore their births, many of these mothers are surprised to realize that in fact they were suppressing parts of the birth experience because they didn't want to dwell on the negatives. It is important to note that there is a difference between dwelling on the negatives and honouring the full experience, which includes feeling *all of it*.

Yes, I struggled with postpartum depression (and depression for years) and much later I expressed the symptoms of post traumatic stress 'disorder' (PTSD). True, I have not been without pain and trauma. However, I couldn't have had traumatic births. I gave birth at home and giving birth at home does not result in birth trauma. *Right?*

Wait. Can you hear the ideology in that statement: 'Giving birth at home does not result in birth trauma?' Really? Is that true? I learned very quickly that this statement is untrue. I have sat with mothers who gave birth at home and who experienced or perceived their births as traumatic.

I am always grateful afterward when I can let go of my biases and widen my gaze. However, the process of elimination is not neat and tidy. In fact, stepping outside of my biases is always met with grief, anguish and internal tension. This is precisely what happened after my birth. My perception of it was skewed because I tried to protect myself, my ideology and my reputation. I was protecting myself from feeling.

What Was I Afraid to Feel

I was ashamed. Or, perhaps more precisely, I was afraid to feel or acknowledge my shame. I was terrified and I was scared to recognize my fear. I experienced regret and I was afraid to feel remorse. I was in extreme pain and I was afraid to touch my grief. I created a wall using what Brené Brown calls the *shame shields*.

I was good at shielding myself from experiencing blame, pain and shame about my childbirth experience. Especially because my identity and reputation was on the line, or so I perceived. I shut down, walled up, hiked up my defense barriers and projected out into the world a story that sounded like this:

> *The birth of my daughter was an unassisted freebirth, which means there were zero caregivers or support persons present aside from the father. It was profoundly empowering and liberating. Even though my daughter had shoulder dystocia and was stuck on my perineum for four contractions and when she was born she did not breathe for a few minutes and that I gave her mouth-to-mouth instinctively. And even though afterwards I contracted a bacterial infection that resulted in hospitalization and two weeks of immobilization with severe abdominal pain and uncontrollable bowel elimination and dehydration. I used to leave out that last part.*

Can you hear the discrepancy in the story? On the one hand, there were aspects of my birth experience that were genuinely otherworldly and profoundly empowering. I never want to diminish this truth. However, if I ignore the other aspects of my birth that were truly filled with moments of terror and fear of death, I would be lying about the impact that this birth had on me.

In the year of 2005, when my daughter was born, I knew nothing about trauma. I was not trauma-informed. I didn't know the signs and symptoms of trauma. As one of my clients recently stated about her birth: I needed to be strong to survive. And this rang true for me as well. I needed to be strong to protect myself, my baby, and my beliefs, so I believed.

In fact, I have needed to appear 'strong'
for nearly two decades now.
Being strong is what I was taught.

Strong meant I did not cry.
Strong meant I did not tire.
Strong said I always put on an I'm okay face.
Strong meant I was not allowed to struggle emotionally.
Strong meant I just kept going and just kept enduring.
Strong meant I could not receive care and rejected medical care that didn't align with my ideology.

Strong meant I suffered physical pain, even excruciating pain.
Strong meant I distanced myself from what I was genuinely feeling
—terror and shame.
Strong meant I put on a front.
Strong meant I NEVER fall apart.

Until one day, YEARS LATER, I fell apart.

The birth of my daughter was a contradiction: I felt incredible power and simultaneously intense terror. This birth tried to crack me open, but I tried not to let it. *I needed to remain strong.* Maybe had I allowed myself to experience grief and terror with compassion I could have protected myself from a future PTSD diagnosis? However, this was not how the story unfolded.

The story I had been telling was not complete because I still had unprocessed emotional material that surfaced each time I told the tale. I would purposely leave out parts because I was protecting myself from pain and judgment.

What I observed is that when I engaged in sharing about my freebirth, I felt uncomfortable. I wanted to hold back or change parts of the story. I often told aspects of the story from a distant perspective; this or that happened, and it was no big deal—that kind of sharing.

**Humans do this: withhold painful points
to protect ourselves from feeling too much.**

A traumatic experience is deemed as such because the event triggers terror, a loss of power and control, and a profound threat to one's sense of safety. All of these things result in the physiological activation of the stress response. As humans, we are not immune to trauma. There will be numerous experiences throughout our lives when we experience a traumatic event. In fact, we are fashioned physiologically to respond to trauma and resolve traumatic material. Thus, we can restore our body back to a state of homeodynamics (a harmonious coherent state of continuous movement).

Not only are we created with such an intelligent system, we are also primed to seek out loving connections with others[3]. Connections help us heal.

---

3   Stephen W Porges, "Love: An Emergent Property of the Mammalian Autonomic Nervous System," *Psychoneuroendocrinology* 23, no. 8 (1998): 837–61, doi:10.1016/S0306-4530(98)00057-2.

On the other hand, unresolved trauma results in the interruption of our primary instinctive drive to connect with love and to foster secure attachment[4].

I realized that I was still holding unprocessed emotional material during a group therapy session I was leading. In this session, a mother shared the unique story of her birthing experience with the group and it hit me all at once. The story she told sounded familiar to my story and awakened me to the aspects of my birth that had been held in the shadows.

A mirror within this mother's story reflected to me, for the first time, that I too had experienced giving birth as traumatic. Since then, I have started telling my true story.

The Birth:
Told Without *Hiding* in Shame

It was 6 a.m. on July 6, 2005, when I woke with a twinge in my uterus. I knew today was the day. My mucous plug released and the aches were frequent. I had my two other children, who were toddlers at the time, picked up that morning and I called my previous husband to return home after having just landed in Toronto for work. Then I went back to sleep and managed to get a deep, restful sleep until the contractions woke me around noon. I remember feeling excited.

I walked into the kitchen, waiting for my husband to return, and I had a feeling I had never experienced with my other two labours—*I was utterly free*. It was the degree of freedom that made me ecstatic. My experience would be self-directed, and no external experts would look at me, measure me, monitor me or tell me how I needed to be. It was glorious and liberating.

My husband arrived with a smoothie in hand around 1 pm and, as soon as he did, I jumped into a birthing pool we had set up in the living room. I remember thinking to myself *I got this, and I know how to give birth*. Labour progressed rapidly and before I knew it I was in the hugeness of the contractions that were taking me on a wild ride. Although familiar, each contraction was rushing through me like a massive wave crashing in on the shore.

There was a moment where I felt torn in half in a way that I didn't remember with my other two births. I recall telling myself in that moment: go deeper, Jennifer. Thankfully, I understood what that meant. I knew that if I took my inner awareness

---

[4] Stephen W. Porges, "The Polyvagal Theory: New Insights into Adaptive Reactions of the Autonomic Nervous System," *Cleveland Clinic Journal of Medicine*, 2009, doi:10.3949/ccjm.76.s2.17; Bonnie Badenoch, *Being a Brain Wise Therapist: A Practical Guide To Interpersonal Neurobiology* (New York, New York: W.W. Norton & Norton, 2008); Mary Main, Erik Hesse, and Siegfried Hesse, "Attachment Theory and Research: Overview with Suggested Applications to Child Custody," *Family Court Review* 49, no. 3 (2011): 426–63, doi:10.1111/j.1744-1617.2011.01383.x; Daniel J Siegel, "Practicing Mindsight" (Sounds True, 2015), https://www.udemy.com/practicing-mindsight/

and attention and directed it towards the intense pain, I could expand and potentially shift the sensation.

I knew that if I allowed the panic to overwhelm me I would reverse the progression of my labour. I knew I needed to find my way through the pain and at this moment to go deeper into the sensations, not away from it. I was grateful for my knowledge and capacity to dive into the enormously painful sensations because what happened next has forever changed my perception and consciousness.

What I 'saw' was otherworldly.
And I hang onto this nugget of gold.

As I directed my attention toward the intensity within my body, I gazed with my inner eye intensely into the pain. I located it in my body. It was within my pelvis structure. Each time the intensity would build, I noticed I wanted to escape the sensation, and thus, I would willfully go deeper into the feeling and pay attention to what was occurring.

And as I did this, I noticed that the sensations changed, and I was pulled into a profound altered state of consciousness. In that state, I saw with my inner eye my pelvis in a 3D fashion. I explored it thoroughly from all angles. It was like I was floating in space with my pelvis.

And then magic happened.

I went into the pelvic bone structure and before my inner eyes, the bony material shifted into dancing molecules. The deeper I went, the more I experienced space between the particles. It was ALL space.

I understood on a cellular level, in that moment of stillness, that what quantum physicists have been saying about the nature of matter and the universe, is in fact true. We are all space and particles dancing together.

I understood that women do not give birth from this physical dimension, but rather we give birth from the plane that quantum physics calls *the field*. Thinking about how babies fit through the birth canal is enough to make anyone feel trepidations about trusting that women's bodies know how to give birth. It is downright terrifying when you think about it. How does something that is bone fit through another object that is also bone and soft tissue?

We cannot give birth from the perspective of 'matter' alone. We must consider another paradigm of possibility. Quantum physics is the science of possibility that teaches us about how the tiniest particles are influenced by a field of energy and information. It made sense to me in that deep state of altered consciousness anything is possible—including giving birth.

Once this awareness hit me, I was catapulted out of my trance-like state and into the downpour of my daughter rushing through my birth canal. Her head was emerging. It was glorious and wild. My body arched and floated in the water and I roared her through my birth canal.

I wish I could stop the story here. Often, *I did*. Up until this point, labour was amazingly empowering and I would never tell it any other way. However, what occurred next is where the trauma set in. As her head crowned, I felt a flood of adrenaline coursing through my veins. Attached to it was fear.

Adrenaline is an important hormone at this stage of labour. It wakes you up and helps to facilitate the final 'fetal ejection' phase of birth. It pumps stress chemicals into the fetus to help 'excite' breathing instincts upon birth. From this point of view, the adrenaline was a 'normal' part of my labour. However, at that point, flashes of her getting stuck ran through my mind - this was my hidden core fear. I knew she was big, but how big I was not sure.

Maybe I knew too much about birth and midwifery, and all that knowledge overwhelmed my psyche? Perhaps I had played out my greatest fear in my mind too many times before my delivery? Maybe deep down inside I didn't want to freebirth but was afraid to reach out for help? Suppose I had intuition about what might present during the birth of my daughter? Or, maybe it had nothing to do with any of that? I will never really know.

> As I held her head and it emerged from my vagina,
> **I felt so much power in my hands.**

I experienced this moment as if I was receiving the power of the cosmos. And when I realized the size of her head, I held my breath. With the next contraction, I waited for her body to be born.

But she didn't budge.

With the following contraction, I flipped onto my hands and knees and waited for her body to be born. Still no movement. My body was full of panic at this stage, as I *knew* that she was stuck and the longer she was sitting on my perineum the higher the risk of oxygen deprivation. I was no longer conscious of the quantum field, I was present to my panic and what was occurring.

I stood up in the pool. I was bewildered and unsure of how I was going to birth my daughter. There were no experts. There were no forceps or vacuums. No one could pull her out. I HAD to birth her. I sensed that I was leaving my body and freezing in fear. Her father took his hands and attempted to help her move her shoulders, but she wouldn't budge.

He looked at me and I caught his gaze. With firmness, he spoke (the only time he talked throughout this entire labour) and said, "Jen, you got this. You are going to push so hard and you are NOT going to stop until she is born."

I nodded, eyes bulging out of my head, and I prayed.

I remember praying to every woman who has gone before me to help me find the power to give birth to my baby. I felt a rush of energy enter my system and I tapped into a wild raging power. I pushed with Olympic force. My daughter flew out of me with a loud pop and dove head first into the waters below. Her father tried to catch her but the force was too much. I spun around and with ninja speed scooped her out of the tub.

She surfaced. And she was flat.

I knew in my heart and soul that she was going to be okay. I called her in. Told her how loved she was. Yet, she had still not taken her first breath. I sucked mucous from her nose with my mouth and I gave her my breath—mouth to mouth. As soon as I did, she opened her eyes. I instructed her to breathe now. Eventually, she took her first breath.

Those minutes felt like eons. I held my breath during that time as we waited. Doubt, terror and shame started to flood my system. Had I done something wrong? Was this all my fault? The words coursed through my being. She was okay. And, she was big. I, however, was flooded with fear.

I went from profound spaciousness to utter terror. I felt fear in all of my body. I tried to talk myself out of the terror. However, it was stuck. I logically knew that newborns can withstand a lack of breath for a few minutes after birth because they are flooded with oxygenated blood cells as they are born. I trusted in physiology. However, I lacked trust in myself and my choices.

PANIC. SHAME. BLAME.

It started to settle into my cells. I lost trust in myself at that moment. My postpartum felt overwhelming. I wanted to be cared for. I wanted a midwife to reassure me that all was well. I had a friend help in the immediate postpartum, but that was not enough. I called a retired midwife and she graciously came to my home and assessed us. I sensed she was a bit worried because of the size of my daughter. She weighed around 10.5 lbs. And I noticed that I was beginning to run a fever.

Things felt blurry in the postpartum. I was shaky. Anticipating the arrival of the after pains to kick in, I was on guard. On day two they kicked in full force and the cramping was utterly horrifying. I didn't remember the after pains being so intense in my previous birth. I couldn't leave my bed, and when the rushes would happen, I was moaning and groaning as if I was in labour again. I started to worry that I had retained pieces of the placenta.

During this time, in the immediate postpartum, I shut out the external world. I was already in defense mode because my family didn't understand my choice to have a freebirth. I needed to pretend I was okay and that everything was just fine. I sensed their fear and concern and I wanted nothing to do with it. Around day 4 postpartum I was hospitalized (time was a bit of a blur). My greatest fear of needing to go to the hospital became a reality.

I had been experiencing explosive diarrhea for a day now, with excruciating abdominal and uterine pain, and I was running a fever. I could not sleep, and at one point I went into a state of convulsion, rocking back and forth on all fours, nursing my newborn, moaning in agony. Yet, I resisted going to the hospital. I was protecting myself from being judged and scolded for the choice I had made. It wasn't until I asked my aunt, who was a nurse, to come over and help me, that I budged. When she arrived and saw me, she told me I needed to go to the hospital immediately. She said I was very sick and dehydrated.

The drive to the hospital was horrific. At this point, time and space were collapsing in on themselves. I was very disoriented. I knew I needed help. When we arrived, I walked in and was admitted. As they took my information and asked me questions, I was scared they would not understand. They were confused about where to 'put' me in the hospital. They needed to know who I 'belonged' to; who they could blame for my state. They asked what happened.

I told them point blank that I chose to birth at home without a caregiver *for religious purposes*. I lied. I am not affiliated with a religious organization and I didn't choose to birth at home alone for religious purposes. I told them that I had a midwife check on me in the postpartum, but that she was not my midwife and was not responsible for me. They wrote down her name and I felt concerned that she was going to get in trouble for having supported me in the postpartum.

I felt guilty. All around.

I asked for morphine and the intern said I could not have it because they did not know what was wrong yet. She said I was severely dehydrated, and my symptoms were akin to Dysentery or Childbed Fever. I liked her. I remember looking deeply into her eyes and trying to send her a message that sounded like, "Please help me. I am in agony. Please be gentle and kind."

The OB/GYN arrived, and he was neither kind nor gentle. He was aggressive with his touch and I screamed out in horror. I asked him to stop touching me, but he wouldn't listen. I felt he was rough with me because he wanted to punish me for my choices. He told me I was experiencing this because of the herbs I had drank. *Whatever*, I remember thinking.

I had not had any vaginal exams with this pregnancy, so having the doctor aggressively examine my fresh and raw birth canal threw me over the edge and I flew entirely out of my body. He also performed a rectal exam without my consent, which left me feeling utterly humiliated.

How can I go from **empowered** to **degraded** so rapidly?

I visualized kicking the doctor in the chest and seeing him fly across the room. But I couldn't do that; I was paralyzed. And so was my husband, as he stood there and watched the scene unfold while holding our newborn daughter.

It was a nightmare. Time had stopped, and I felt like I was in a horror movie. I rapidly took in two bags of saline solution to rehydrate. After running a few tests, they were unable to determine what was wrong with me. I knew what was wrong with me: *I contracted a bacterial infection from the pool* (more on that in a moment). They wanted to put me in quarantine, without my daughter, until they knew what was going on.

I said no.

They didn't give me antibiotics because they didn't know if they would work. So, I left the next day, after 24 hours in the hospital, against their wishes. What followed was a two-week recovery phase and more shame.

When I got home, I was bedridden, and I had no control of my bowels for close to two weeks. I was humiliated as I laid on a diaper because mucous was oozing out of my rectum. All I did was nurse, sleep, and drink tea and smoothies. I had a large community of support and an angel mother figure who came and sat at my head for hours in the evening, holding me and sending energy in silence. These moments were grace-filled. However, I could not feel gratitude. I was stuck in terror and protection mode.

As I write, I realize now how many people came to my side and offered counsel, support, nourishment and love. And how I need to reach out to them and thank them for all they had provided. Without them, I am not sure I would have pulled through.

> I was loved. However, I couldn't feel love.

This is a result of trauma. According to Porges, when we are in survival, our capacity to love and to being loved is compromised[5]. And when we are in a shame response, we cannot access empathy for ourselves or others.

Eventually my health returned, albeit slowly. I struggled with how long it took to regain my energy. I was impatient with it all because I was supposed to be with my midwifery cohort, studying together, in the US. I wanted to be there with my newborn, not struggling for my life and health.

I felt totally fractured.

I stored parts of my birth as traumatic memories in my mind and body. And, I internalized the experience as such:

I did something wrong.
It was all my fault.
I made a stupid choice.
I should have known better.
I could have died.
My baby could have died.
I can't trust my body.
I am too radical.
I don't deserve to be happy.
I don't deserve loving care.
I am bad.

These statements were deeply embedded in my subconscious and became the internalized perceptions associated with the birth of my daughter. They became the associated channels that were wired to a neural network of information about the birth of my daughter. The undercurrent of these statements resulted in a deep sense of shame and failure, with a core belief being that *I am bad*.

Shame is the most disempowering feeling we experience. Shame is internalized as an *I am* statement. It's about me, myself and I. Whereas guilt is a result of focusing on behavior—*I made a mistake*—it is not about *being* bad or wrong. Shame debilitates. When we are living in the shame mode, we activate our defenses.

---

[5] Porges, "The Polyvagal Theory: New Insights into Adaptive Reactions of the Autonomic Nervous System," 2009.

NO ONE WANTS TO BE SEEN IN THEIR SHAME.

I didn't want anyone to know that I was deeply ashamed of my birth choice. Even though I was in traumatic pain, shame won. There was no room for compassion. Just an internal drive to survive or, more profound yet, a drive to prove myself. I could not be wrong. So, began the big lie. The lie emerged because I was afraid to explore my shame.

I was scared to be vulnerable.
I was afraid to be seen.
I was afraid to face my pain.
I was fearful of receiving love and care.
I was scared to look honestly at my birth
I was scared to hold it all in a place of loving kindness and reflection.

What if freebirth was dangerous? Or wrong? Or too radical?
What if I did decide to freebirth out of a place of extremes and fear?
What if I could have prevented my daughter from being stuck?
What if I could have prevented my sickness?
What if... What if... What if...

Swarming with what ifs, I was overwhelmed with uncomfortable emotions. Instead of processing the traumatic material, digesting and feeling it, I walled up. I was a rock. No one could reach me, and my defenses were activated.

I engaged in the worst fight ever with my mother during that time. It nearly destroyed our relationship. My mother almost chose to remove herself from my life because she was in so much pain watching me suffer and be confused about my state and choices. I was ready to stand alone, to defend my decision. All in an attempt to keep myself from feeling shame.

As I write, I feel the well of sadness emerge again in my chest and throat. I see how much pain my postpartum-self was in. How tormented she was. How terrified she was. And how frozen she was.

My healing work is not finished. I recognize that the creation of the Healing After Birth program, the passion for understanding trauma, the training to work with trauma and heal, and the compassion I experience each day for mothers, is in part my preparation to help facilitate deep healing.

We heal together. Collectively.

Our stories course through each other, lifting the stones weighing heavy from our past births, so we can have the courage to heal. My courage to share the fullness of my story and acknowledge that my healing is still alive could not have been possible had I not sat in witness of other mothers' stories.

And, as I mentioned earlier, one story in particular awoke an implicit memory associated with my birth. I am grateful for this awakening. I will not tell my story differently anymore in an attempt to protect myself or others from the shocking details. I will tell my birth story without shame and blame. It is the only way I can genuinely integrate the experience as part of my medicine.

SHAME IS AT THE CRUX OF OUR INABILITY TO HEAL

Shame keeps us paralyzed. Shame creates the mask that we put on for others. Shame is the monster we don't want to look at. I know now that I no longer need to hold onto my shame. And my healing will continue to happen alongside you, as we walk together into the muddy waters of birth trauma.

Each story is unique just like each birth experience is unique. It is not a competition. Healing is not a competition about who's trauma is more real. As I tell my story, you may recognize aspects of your story. Whether you wanted a hospital birth, home birth, birth center birth or unassisted birth, your experience is valid. Regardless of how it turned out, your experience is valid.

There is no such thing as *not traumatic enough*. You don't need to fear that no one will relate or that you don't belong. I felt all those things. I felt isolated and alone with my internal anguish. However, now I'm here to help dismantle the walls of separation that many of us with trauma experience. I honestly believe the late Jeannine Parvati Baker's comment that, *"as we heal birth, we heal the earth"*, is truth.

As we heal our wounded birth stories, we heal our wounded connections with our self and others. Healing awakens a newfound capacity to love. And love heals.

CHAPTER 2

SETTING THE STAGE FOR HEALING

Foundational Needs for Recovery and Healing

Judith Herman, a pioneer within the field of trauma recovery, recognized that women with histories of domestic violence and abuse were suffering from PTSD and that trauma was not just reserved for war veterans or those who suffered environmental catastrophe[6].

With this in mind, Herman outlined a three-phased approach to trauma recovery. This approach has been taken into consideration and incorporated throughout this guidebook. The three phases are: Establishing safety and building tolerance, working with the traumatic material, and the final phase is integration[7]

Foundationally, humans need the following to support wellbeing and encourage integration of stressful events:

- ★ A safe and secure environment.
- ★ People who respond with a calm, connected, and attuned presence.
- ★ A capacity to tolerate stressful material in their body.
- ★ A capacity to experience strong emotional information.
- ★ An environment that fosters love and connection.
- ★ A freedom to express one's spiritual beliefs.

---

6   Judith L Herman, "Review of Special Issue: Guidelines for Treating Dissociative Identity Disorder in Adults (3rd Revision); Rebuilding Shattered Lives: Treating Complex PTSD and Dissociative Disorders; and Understanding and Treating Dissociative Identity Disorder: A Relati," *Psychoanalytic Psychology* 29, no. 2 (2012): 267–69, doi:10.1037/a0027818; Simington, Trauma Recovery Certification Handbook.

7   Judith Herman, *Trauma and Recovery*, 2nd ed. (New York: Perseus Book Group, 1997).

Every human has different strengths and vulnerabilities that impact their capacity to tolerate highly stressful events. As such, Judith noted that before any form of integration of one's traumatic experiences can occur, establishing safety is foundational.

Therefore, we will begin by focusing on cultivating safety with both the internal and external environment being taken into consideration. Your internal environment includes everything that occurs *behind* the mind's eye. The external environment includes people, places and things. All of which can also be spoken as your internal reality and your external reality.

Establishing Safety and Creating Containment

Before embarking upon any trek, you must assess for safety. Without safety, the nervous system signals an alert that results in the activation of stress responses. I am not talking only about physical safety, but also emotional and mental safety. Within the field of trauma therapy, before the client and therapist dive into deep matters, both need to ensure that the client:

* ★ feels safe
* ★ has a good report
* ★ understands the terrain
* ★ is committed to the process
* ★ can swim and knows how to get herself to the shore lines if need (i.e. can regulate her emotional system if she feels overwhelmed)
* ★ can tolerate a fair amount of emotional and mental material without dissociating or becoming overly dysregulated

A simple yet effective method to establish safety is simply to scan your environment and assess it. Take in your surroundings and tell yourself: *In this moment, I am safe*. If for some reason your environment is unsafe, it is critical to find a safe space before proceeding. As such, your nervous system will not relax. Rather, it will remain in high alert, in preparation to react to a potential threat.

You cannot heal if you are stuck in high alert.

That said, one of the symptoms of trauma is being stuck in hypervigilance – always on defense and feeling hyperaware. This state of being is exhausting and the goal is to shift out of hypervigilance and into a state of calm, even if for just a few minutes. Training your system to recognize 'real' threats vs 'perceived' threats is key.

In an activated trauma state, the system cannot differentiate between the two. Thus, telling your system – your biological body – that there are no threats or predators in the room at this time, while scanning with your eyes all corners of your space, can help train the system to trust that statement.

Before you begin, go ahead scan and assess your environment.
Take a moment to notice what is happening within your body and mind.
Is your system activated? What does that feel like?
Is your system calming down? What does that feel like?
At any moment throughout the day, if you feel activated, you can scan for safety and remind your system that you are safe in this moment (if you truly are).

Another effective and important tool you can use to calm an activated or aroused system is the *butterfly hug*. Go ahead and Google 'butterfly hug' or 'tapping for anxiety'. You will find some tutorials that outline how to use bi-lateral tapping for calming and integrating stressful material. The best part is that you can teach this to your kids when they get overstimulated with big sensations in their bodies.
 There a few more effective tools that will help you work with those big feelings and sensations you experience in your body. The next suggestion is so obvious, but in moments of panic and overwhelm, we forget about it.

The simple breath.
 Follow your breath. Notice your breath. Stay with your breath. Find your breath. Watch your breath. The breath will help you find your way through. It is a guiding force in and of itself. When we are overly charged with stressful material, we forget about our breath, and often do not want to 'be with the breath'. Being with the breath means that we have to feel what is going on. However, the breath is our friend, not our enemy. I encourage you to take a breath. Right now. Just be with your breath and begin to notice what you experience in your body and mind.
 So far, all the examples have been things you can do individually, but we heal collectively and in fact, we learn how to regulate our nervous system in relation to another person or mammal. **This is called co-regulating.** Finding a person, therapist or healer who can hold an attuned calm state while you are highly activated, will entrain your system to their system. What does this mean? It means that there is an invisible energetic connection occurring between the two people. Based on entrainment theory and entanglement theory, the person with the strongest and calmest frequency will influence the other frequency in the room. If the person holding the space has a cohesive and calm frequency, and the other is dysregulated, the calm cohesive vibration is stronger because it is coherent, therefore, it will influence the state of the other frequencies present.

Have you heard the statement: *The strongest frequency in the room has the most power?* I do not recall who said this first; however, I do know this to be true. I believe that it is the act of presence that makes therapy effective—that which is invisible and cannot be measured using standard tools.

This is why choosing *who* holds your space and story is critically important; they need to be able to hold a stronger coherent frequency so that your system can learn how to regulate itself.

Who comes to mind? Anyone?

When you consider therapy from this perspective, does it feel less intimidating? The idea that those who are going to help you heal your nervous system are not necessarily analyzing you for all your faults, but rather collaborating with you to help teach your system how to be and remain calm.

Finally (but not limited to), I want to highlight the importance of **grounding techniques** as another tool to consider. What does it mean to ground? The best way to describe grounding is to imagine that there are roots growing out of your feet and that they are anchored deep into the earth. You know that your body is here, on the ground, connected to matter. You establish a sense of knowing where you begin and end. When we are activated by traumatic memory or material, sometimes we lose contact with our bodies, self, and surroundings. Grounding helps to restore this disconnected state.

Grounding can help in the following ways:
- ★ Bring you back into your center.
- ★ Help you get back into your body.
- ★ Help you calm down an activated nervous system response.
- ★ Help you think and see clearly.
- ★ Help you integrate physiological trauma.
- ★ Help you 'feel' felt sensations in your body.
- ★ Increase capacity to stay with those 'sensations'.
- ★ Help you identify emotions.
- ★ Help you stay present with what is occurring.

Tools to help with grounding:
- ★ We can ground using our breath.
- ★ We can ground using mental imagery (e.g., trees or safe place).
- ★ We can ground by moving our body (e.g., dancing or yoga).
- ★ We can ground by walking on the earth barefooted.

What other ways can you ground?

To deepen your healing experience, you are invited to apply to the ***Healing After Birth Program*** in which you will receive 6 one-on-one sessions PLUS weekly videos, audios, guided meditations, and therapeutic activities. If you are not ready to engage with this level of therapeutic support, you can sign up for a BONUS audio to support inner resourcing and connecting to your calm place. Both intended to help you feel supported and held as you dive into healing your birth experience. Head on over to www.jennifersummerfeldt.com and click on 'FREE Audio' link to access the audio files.

REFLECTIVE EXERCISE
ON SAFETY & GROUNDING

Why do you need to practice grounding?

What do you already do to ground and centre yourself?
How do you know when you are being activated/triggered?

What do you already do to foster safety?

How do you calm down when you feel overwhelmed?
What helps?

What do you already know about your capacity to tolerate big feelings and sensations within your body?

CHAPTER 3

UNDERSTANDING SHAME

Motherhood and Shame

>Don't co-sleep; do co-sleep.

>Don't birth at home; birth at home.

>Don't work outside the home; go back to work.

>Breast is best; it's okay to bottle feed.

>Too much screen time; no screen time.

>Vaginal birth; choose a Caesarean.

>Let them cry; don't let them cry.

>Vaccinate; don't vaccinate.

Each day we are bombarded with opinions about how to give birth and raise our children. From the moment we plan to conceive or find ourselves surprisingly pregnant, a whole new world opens. For many, entering the world of motherhood for the first time is like walking through a vortex. On one side of this invisible shield lives all the mothers who have gone before us, and on the other side is the world 'out there'.

Let's agree that there is a world unto itself that is not visible or understandable until you have been initiated into the 'tribe' called motherhood. Pregnancy is the first phase of initiation in which we learn, rather quickly, that our bodies become the gawk and opinion of strangers and 'experts'. In addition, for many first-time mothers, growing another human inside of our wombs is a strange experience that can for some, feel 'alien' and foreign. somehow, we are supposed to love and connect and take care of this growing embryo.

The doubt sets in early. is my body strong enough, healthy enough and capable of bearing children? The shame starts early too. let's explore some of the areas where it can show up throughout the childbearing years.

Prenatal Shame

Many women experience shame if they miscarry or are challenged to conceive. Often left unsupported and silenced throughout these experiences, it is a rare woman who doesn't think that her body failed them and that they are somehow defective. And for those who 'get' pregnant, the worry sets in deep.

Will my body hold onto this one?

The famous Brené Brown, on vulnerability and shame, shares that shame is an emotion attached to our core beliefs – I am bad/defective/wrong . Whereas, guilt is an emotion connected to the mindset that I have done something – I have made a mistake/done something wrong/done something bad.

You can hear and feel the difference between these two challenging emotions—guilt and shame: shame focuses on a belief that 'you are flawed' whereas guilt focuses on a belief that 'you did something wrong'. Neither guilt nor shame are comfortable emotions to feel. However, there is a sense that with guilt, you can do something about the situation—you can change it or make it better or learn from the mistake. Whereas, with shame, you become debilitated by it and there is a sense that it/you cannot be changed. At such a core level, the shameful beliefs define who you are (even if they are untrue).

Childbirth Shame

Back to motherhood. If women did not experience shame about their bodies failing them prenatally, many will experience shame about their bodies throughout the delivery. This shame sounds like: I couldn't give birth vaginally, I tried for hours but my body wouldn't progress. I just wouldn't go into labour. I tried everything, and nothing worked. I wouldn't stop bleeding. I didn't have room for my baby to fit in my pelvis. My baby was in the wrong position (and it was my fault due to my lifestyle). I just couldn't give birth. The experts knew best. And so on.

> Underneath each of these statements are the core beliefs that
> **my body is flawed, I am flawed, I failed, I am a failure,
> I did it wrong, I am wrong, my body is broken, I am broken.**

Mothers protect themselves from feeling shame. This is instinctive. We are motivated to move away from pain. Shame produces an enormous amount of emotional pain. Shame produces more shame, and the cycle repeats itself, feeding off each shameful belief like a hungry ghost.

> *It is impossible to thrive in motherhood
> if the underpinning of becoming a mother is founded in shame.*

I want to highlight that this motherhood shame voice is not an individually personal voice, but rather a collective voice that has infiltrated and been imprinted into our psyches due to a dominant cultural worldview that devalues the mother, and for centuries, woman's work (more on this later). Let's keep unpacking shame.

Postpartum Shame

Let's explore the next opportunity for mothers to experience shame. If shame did not present during labour and birth, it can rear its nasty head in the postpartum. All of a sudden, a woman magically becomes a mother and is expected to know how to raise this human being. Most mothers are afraid of 'fucking up' and 'ruining their child/ren'. There is a lot of pressure to 'do it right'. This poses the question: what is 'right' parenting anyways?

The pressure appears immediately after the birth in that mothers are expected to know how to breastfeed. Women's boobs are grabbed, pinched and yanked in an attempt to 'get the baby to latch'. There is so much stress focused on the act of breastfeeding that even if the birth went as planned, mothers feel anxious about not being able to breastfeed. Again, denoting one's worth as a mother.

Breastfeeding, at the deepest level, signifies the mother's ability to nourish her child. There is a huge psychological hurdle one must go through if they cannot, or choose not to, breastfeed. Somewhere deep within the psyche there is a worry (shared collectively) that if I cannot nourish my baby, i am somehow defective. And from a survival point of view, my baby could die. Even if this is not conscious, you can imagine the amount of stress a mother would feel to ensure that her baby is nourished.

If there is any indication that she may not be able to nurse her baby—not enough milk, difficult latch, baby losing weight, tongue tie, colic—she will often be quick to move towards formula feeding to mitigate any risk of malnourishment. Thankfully, because of technological advancements and food production, we can ensure that our babies will be fed.

However, this does not address the fact that many mothers feel devastated and devalued as a mother if they cannot breastfeed. Once again, pointing towards the shameful core belief—I am defective/I am a bad mother. When does a new mother have the time to focus on these deeper core beliefs and debilitating emotions?

Time takes on a new meaning in motherhood. Time warps. Days turn into nights, and nights turn into days. This changing time schedule is a challenge for many modern mothers to adjust to. This gives rise to sleep deprivation and another layer of shameful perceptions that sounds like: my baby won't sleep through the night (and this is a reflection of my parenting), i can't sleep, there is something wrong with me, I can only sleep with my baby (and this is shunned by friends and family, so I am a bad mother), I can't sleep when my baby is next to me, so they sleep in a crib (and this is shunned by friends and family, so I am a bad mother).

Shame displays its ugly face every turn of the way as a mother; it is merely impossible to avoid it.

I have not yet touched on the topic of postpartum mood disorders (PPMD). Lately my sense is that more women fear PPMD than fear childbirth. To begin, I would like to rephrase the term 'mood disorders' to that of 'postpartum mood and mental unrest'. Where did the notion that the postpartum period would be smooth sailing come from? That somehow our lives would not be turned upside down and inside out?

My sense is that, generally speaking, mothers are surprised by the immense and intense changes and challenges experienced throughout the postpartum phase. I hear mothers say that they spent all their energy preparing for the birth and had no idea that motherhood would be so hard.

I think we have glorified pregnancy, like a cool hip trendy idea that comes with new gadgets and wearing apparatuses. We have glorified the image of the beautiful good mother, who is smiling and engaged, and has it all together. And we have failed to be realistic about the harsh truth about transitioning into motherhood – conception, pregnancy, birth, postpartum are all initiatory events, that cannot be avoided, in preparation for motherhood.

So, we are left with an either/or mentality, striving for something unrealistically portrayed by pop-culture. If we experience anything less than the glorified image of motherhood, we are left to silently question our role as a mother as not being good enough.

> The ultimate failure for women who have children is to fail as a mother.

There is both an external and an internal burden to perfect motherhood. Because anything less would/could result in 'messing up' our kids. And to live with the knowing that our children have suffered because of us, as mothers, is almost unbearable to experience. Thus, we avoid feeling our shame, questioning our assumptions, and transforming our beliefs because we want to create a buffer between day-to-day reality and the paralyzing feelings we might experience.

From my perspective, when we avoid getting to the nitty gritty of our shame, we live from a place of chronic anxiety and/or depression (deep insecurity and unrest). And, from this place we are motivated to fill the void, contain the painful aches within and silence the 'not good enough' voice with external 'stuff'. We consume anything that will offer a moment of comfort and hope including wine, ideas, courses, activities, food, sex, more kids, Netflix, etc. You get the idea.

> We look outside of ourselves to find the answers
> that can only be found by going within.

Shame pushes us to our edges, to our limits. Fostering a chronic self-image of worthlessness. If we have not been shown how to be with our shame and transform it, it can feel like a daunting and terrifying task. And it seems that very few mothers escape motherhood without feeling shame.

Just the other night, my maternal grandmother spoke about all the ways she failed as a mother. How today's mothers have more help, resources and knowledge about how to be a 'good mother'. And how she wishes she could do it all over again. She was choking back her tears, as she spoke.

On the surface, it may appear that modern mothers have all the answers and resources at their fingertips, and yet, I would argue that the pain of motherhood still exists in full force. It's probably even more complicated because we are expected to be more self-aware nowadays and many of us are not in survival mode in the same ways that our pioneering foremothers experienced.

Generally speaking, today's Western mother has access to more resources, more knowledge, more supportive partners and more money than our western foremothers and yet there is still shame. Why is that?

Because shame is an imprint.

Let me explain. Our natural state is not one of shame. One might argue that our natural state is of love and compassion. Shame is a patterned response to stressful and adverse circumstances. It is hard to imagine that shame has any productive purpose except to keep us small and insignificant.

I can't help but think that patriarchy is one reason why women feel small and believe that we as mothers/woman are insignificant. In order for patriarchy to survive and thrive, women need to believe that they are inadequate, defective and 'crazy'. Within western civilization, there is a patriarchal worldview. This cannot be argued. And we have been trying to fit 'motherhood' and 'womanhood' into this perceptual lens. It has not been easy.

We are imprinted by both the dominant societal beliefs, and our family of origin's historical beliefs and experiences. What if the shameful voice that is experienced as being real and yours/mine does not belong to you? What if you were taught to feel ashamed for generations. Taught to be ashamed about your body, your gender, your sexuality, and yes, about motherhood. What we may be experiencing today, is a result of a belief system that is systemic and intergenerational. What if it (shame) is bigger than you and outside of you, but not you?

We now know that when the fetus is developing within the mother's womb, the mother downloads information about the world via chemical transactions to the fetus's nervous system. How the mother internalizes stress, trauma and adversities in life directly impacts how the baby experiences the world and tolerates stressful circumstances.

Yes, I know this sounds like 'mother shaming'. Like somehow it is the mother's fault if you came in with an imprint of your mother's shame. So, we blame our mothers for 'fucking us up'. But wait, how far back can you go? What about her mother? And the foremothers of your lineage? And what about the environment that they were living in? Where does the 'shame' imprint take root? Has it ever been safe to be a woman or a mother? This is a deep wound. The wound I am referring to is the *mother wound.*

(Yes, the paternal figure impacts the child as well, but not through direct chemical transference of stress hormones.)

I am no historian. I cannot recount the history of woman with accuracy. I was not in the department of women's studies while attending post-secondary school, but I have been 'studying' women over the past 20 years as lived experience. My overall sense, based on stories I have heard throughout the years and the imprint I hold as a woman, is that for centuries patriarchy as a global force, has reigned with an agenda to silence and destroy women's instinctive powers. To be clear, patriarchy is the system in which we live within, it does not refer to men in general.

How do we get imprinted with shame?

Let's paint a picture: a baby is developing in the womb and its nervous system, which includes the skull brain, heart brain, gut brain and skin, is being encoded with survival level hormones. The mother is directly informing and imprinting the baby's nervous system. And that mother is being informed by her environment, both immediate and extended. This includes and is not limited to: culture, religion, beliefs, geography, family of origin history, race, and the dominant worldview at that time.

As a biological being, we need this information downloaded throughout our system so that we are prepared to survive within our environment. Once we are born, we are in a symbiotic (enmeshed) relationship with our primary care givers. We experience what our primary care givers experience during this primary period (roughly up to age 2). Throughout the first six-years of our life, we are in an altered-state of consciousness. This allows our brain to absorb information from the environment, and all of that information is stored in the sub-conscious areas of the of our brain (giving rise to the 'autopilot').

We feel and interpret the world through the experiences of our primary caregivers. All of this is communicated via something called mirror neurons. Our primary care givers are 'encoding' or informing our brain about the world we live in. As primarily social beings, we *need* them to help us make sense out of the world and to feel safe.

Ideally, we want to be raised in an environment where we are loved, nourished and attuned to by our primary care givers. But this is rarely the case (however, more of us are working really hard to make this a reality). So instead, we need to learn how to handle stressful circumstances and adversities. *This gives rise to resilience.* How our primary care givers tolerate and integrate adversities imprints our nervous system with either a healthy adaptive stress response or a dysregulated response.

Unfortunately though, generally speaking, few people have been taught how to respond to stressful circumstances in an adaptive manner. If your mother and the women within your family of origin were not given the opportunity to heal their own 'mother wound', then you can assume that shame has been passed onto you.

Furthermore, the way your mother and foremothers made sense out of their adversities may have given rise to a shameful state of being that most likely sounds similar to your internal dialogue.

I call this internal dialogue the 'shame voice'.

For example: I can't do anything right. My body is disgusting and a disgrace. My body is broken. I am a terrible horrible mother. I am insignificant as a woman. I do not matter. I am unlovable. I am bad. I am a failure as a person. My voice doesn't matter. Nothing I do is good enough. I am wrong.

Can you relate to any of these statements? Do they sound familiar?

The fact that you might be able to relate to these statements means that the voice of shame isn't an isolated way of thinking and feeling. It is a collective way of thinking and believing. It exists in the collective mind, not just 'your' mind. In other words, you are not battling this alone, and yet, shame isolates and makes us feel utterly alone in our dark thoughts and lack of worth.

Now what? What is happening for you as you consider the notion that:
  a. The voice of shame is an imprint; and
  b. It is a shared collective experience?

Taking into consideration the proposed notion that we are imprinted by our maternal lineage and that we have a shared intergenerational shame voice, how do we change it? It feels so real and debilitating and gives rise to much of the mental unrest we experience as women and mothers, and yet, it seems impossible to imagine living without shame.

What if we longer believed the shame voice?

Easier said than done. I know. I was totally debilitated by my shame voice for years and I am still working with it. Everywhere we turn there is evidence to suggest that our shame voice is real. We can list a thousand reasons why we should be ashamed.

For example: I yelled at my kids, I left my baby to cry it out, I wanted to throw my baby across the room, I can't stop crying, I didn't want my baby, I can't breastfeed, I am depressed, I didn't want to give birth etc.

> It is not the statement alone that produces a shame response,
> it is what we believe about ourselves in response
> to these circumstances that triggers shame.

I yelled in rage at my kids, I couldn't take it anymore...
  and what does that mean about me as a person?
I left my baby to cry it out...
  and what does that mean about me as a person?

I wanted to throw my baby across the room...
    and what does that mean about me as a person?
I didn't want my baby...
    and what does that mean about me as a person?
I couldn't give birth the way I planned...
    and what does that mean about me as a person?
I can't breastfeed...
    and what does that mean about me as a person?
I had a hard time conceiving...
    and what does that mean about me as a person?
I kept miscarrying...
    and what does that mean about me as a person?

Most often we can trace it to our core beliefs such as: I am a bad mother. I am wrong. I am defective. I am worthless. I am insignificant and inadequate. I am a disgrace. I am unlovable. What are some alternative perspectives that may give rise to a more balanced response?

I yelled at my kids in rage because I was overwhelmed and all alone. I snapped in a moment of weakness because I didn't know an alternative, and my family yelled at me, and now in retrospect I can see that I made a mistake. I am allowed to make mistakes. I am going to take a look at what is challenging for me and see if I can get extra support. In the end, I am doing my best given the circumstances I am in, and I will try and change that which I can change.

I hope I have taken you on a spiraling and winding journey into the concept of motherhood and shame. I raised some deep perspectives and acknowledge that I only touched the surface of many of these statements. My hope is that something within these pages has ignited a desire to explore more, question more, and heal more.

Most importantly, that you walk away having heard:

You are not alone in your shame.
Shame is not uniquely yours, it is a shared worldview.
Healing and changing your core beliefs is possible.

REFLECTIVE EXERCISE
ON SHAME

Do you carry shameful thoughts or perceptions about your birth or your role as a mother? If yes, what does that voice sound like? What do you hear yourself say to yourself?

Where do you feel shame in your body?

How does shame show up? How does it disempower you? What happens?

Personify your 'shame voice'. Give it a name, a character, a description. Who and what is it? What does it look like? Where does it live? How familiar is it? How long have you had it for? When was it born?

Is shame preventing you from healing? If so, how?

THERAPEUTIC ACTIVITY
NARRATIVE EXERCISE

This activity encourages you to explore your feelings associated with the shadow of shame. You just learned a lot about the internal voice of shame and how it may be showing up for you. I invite you to consider the following question and engage in the art of letter writing. After considering the statement below, allow a conversation to flow between 'you' and your voice of shame.

When I think about my relationship to the voice of shame and how it is showing up in my postpartum, I would like my shame voice to hear the following:

Dear Voice of Shame,

CHAPTER 4

UNDERSTANDING TRAUMA

A New Understanding About Trauma and Childbirth Trauma

Trauma shows up in day-to-day life in the following ways:
- ★ Creating a disconnect from your core self.
- ★ Preventing a connection to your present-day reality.
- ★ Shaping how your mind perceives reality.
- ★ Impairing brain function.
- ★ Dysregulating the nervous system by triggering a state of constant defense and activation (survival mode).
- ★ Distorting and compromising your relationships.
- ★ Producing inflammation throughout the body and decreasing immune function.
- ★ Making it difficult to process emotions and creating erratic and irrational emotional responses.

The 'Coles Notes' on Trauma

Trauma is the expressed physiological, neurological, psychological, relational and spiritual symptoms that resulted from having endured a stressful, violating, horrifying, and/or life-threatening event, in which any sense of safety and wellbeing was shattered.

Trauma is what happens inside of you as a result of the stressful event. Further, both the event itself and the perception of the event must be considered when assessing for and treating trauma. Simply stated, trauma is the end result of having experienced an overwhelmingly stressful event (toxic stress) that was perceived as a threat to your wellbeing or to the wellbeing of your loved ones.

It is important to note that childbirth is a naturally stressful event; however, if at any point you perceived a threat to yourself or your baby, for whatever reason, and you felt trapped and unable to escape the 'danger', your nervous system most likely responded with an activated threat/stress response.

Two people can experience the same event and be impacted differently. Although the event itself is not necessarily traumatic, albeit threatening, the trauma is the result of having experienced the threat. According to Peter Levine, a pioneering expert in trauma, certain events can trigger a traumatic stress response such as: accidents and injury, abuse and attacks, environmental catastrophe, war, severe neglect, malnourishment, surgery, severe illness and childbirth, to name a few.

A few things occur during a traumatic episode:
- ⋆ Your body responds to the threat by releasing chemicals that offer support for you to either fight, flee or freeze in an attempt to grasp for safety (adrenaline and cortisol).
- ⋆ Your mind freezes the experience and links associated thoughts, senses, emotions, and sensations to that experience. This gives rise to the notion in neuroscience that 'what fires together, wires together'.
- ⋆ Then, after the event, people tell themselves something about the event itself. This gives rise to the narrative and internal dialogue.

Due to the fact that our brain is a meaning-making living organism, it seeks to make sense out of the traumatic event. The brain tries to sort through all of the dysregulated material and store it properly as long-term episodic memory.

However, when there is a ton of adrenaline flooding the system because the stress/threat response has been activated (akin to full-throttle gas), the body responds by pumping cortisol into the system in attempt to put out the fires, so to speak (akin to putting on the breaks).

What neuroscience tells us is that when we have too much adrenaline and cortisol in the system, parts of the brain responsible for sorting out the material and storing the information (the hippocampus) is compromised. This means that the emotional centre known as the limbic system (that houses the amygdala, hypothalamus, and the hippocampus) is running the show with erratic, undigestible emotional information.

The emotional centre or the mammalian brain, communicates primarily with the right hemisphere of the brain. This part of the brain is known as our intuitive, creative, spacious, imaginal, expansive, non-linear hemisphere. To learn more about the hemispheres, I encourage you to watch Ian McGilchrist's YouTube RSA explanation of the two hemispheres.

Within the limbic system there is another small part of the brain called the hippocampus. This area is responsible for creating context from the emotional material. Without context the emotional material is all over the place and disorienting.

Trauma compromises the communication between these two parts of the brain (along with other parts as well), therefore the event remains stuck in the realm of dysregulated emotional material, with no context. As such, there is often a feeling that your emotions are in charge, and you are chasing after them, trying to put out the fires.

> Hence, it is imperative to remind yourself that although you may feel all sorts of feelings and emotions, **you are not your emotions.**

Part of the healing process is to discharge the energy of the stress response that is trapped within your system and support all parts of the brain to regain communication so that your emotional system can calm down.

I have met with many mothers who are stuck in high alert and who are overly emotional and feel totally out of control. This is called *dysregulation*. Dysregulation of the system simply means that all the parts of the nervous system, which include the three skull brains, the spinal cord, the gut brain and the heart brain (more on that later) are not in harmony or coherence.

There is a sense that the body is running the show and that you have no control to do anything about it. When this is happening, your body is literally acting as your mind, in that your conscious mind is not in the driver's seat. I often hold the image as if my 'animal suite', aka the body, is running in front of me and my conscious mind (ethereal in nature) is chasing after it. I find this image hilarious when I am sitting in meditation with it; however, in actuality, it is a painful reality for so many of us—leading to chronic exhaustion, disempowerment and a belief that everything is outside of our realm of control. When my nervous system was stuck in high gear, I felt like I was losing my mind.

Some of the symptoms people can experience are:
- Difficulty communicating thoughts.
- Difficulty remembering.
- Uncontrollable rage and anger.
- Uncontrollable sadness.
- Irrational emotional outbursts.
- Difficulty sleeping.
- Nightmares.
- Hypervigilance and alertness (always on guard).

- ★ Avoidance behaviours especially as it pertains to the event.
- ★ Disconnection from others and baby.
- ★ Disembodiment (ungrounded), like floating.
- ★ Difficulty hearing or seeing.
- ★ Feeling trapped in memories.
- ★ Hallucinations.

The Three Broad Categories of Trauma Symptoms

1. Re-experiencing and reliving
This can show up as flashbacks, a sense of being stuck in the scene, always thinking about the event, nightmares, frozen in time. Sometimes, you may not notice these sensations until you are triggered or activated by something (e.g. driving by the hospital). For some, they start to relive the experience when they are pregnant with their next child.

2. Avoiding/constricting
We all do this when we don't want to feel or see something – we avoid looking at it or going to those places that make us feel uncomfortable. Resistance is so common that you may not even realize you are constricting or resisting 'feeling' the pain of the event. As mentioned above, many mothers avoid driving near the hospital for fear of 'feeling too much'. What are you avoiding? What are you resisting? Remember that constricting is a form of protection. It is not bad, it is instinctive. However, in order for healing to take place, letting go of the resistance is key.

3. Arousal/anxiety
Arousal is the symptom that is most often noted. You experience a rapid heart rate, panic, overwhelm, feelings of always being on guard or high alert, lack of sleep, restlessness, irritability, quick to rage or cry and unsettled. The notion of 'calm' feels out of reach.

As you can see, trauma is multifaceted.

One of the pioneers in the field is Dan Siegel, MD. He has written extensively on what he calls Interpersonal Neurobiology and the impact that trauma has on the brain and all its parts, including the mind and relationships. Further, he speaks about how we heal, what fosters mental health, and what promotes integration and encourages coherence.

It is important to note that trauma impacts all aspects of one's life and disconnects people from the essence of being alive. As primarily a social species, one of the deepest pains from trauma is the fractures in one's capacity to bond socially, especially as it pertains to our children and loved ones.

According to Stephen Porges and the Polyvagal Theory, trauma compromises the flow and function of the vagal system, the third branch within the autonomic nervous system, which is responsible for social bonding instincts. I want to highlight this finding because one of the most common concerns I hear from mothers is their difficulty connecting and bonding with their newborn.

Many mothers carry an enormous amount of grief pertaining to this experience and it is important to note that, for the most part, the lack of bonding is physiological not a lack of love or conscious rejection.

Let's pause for a moment.
As you consider this above point, notice how you feel.
What sensations are occurring within your body?
What thoughts are swirling around?

The Impact of Trauma on Childbirth and Bonding

When your body is overwhelmed by an influx of stress chemicals, your instinctive vagal response, which supports the release of the hormone oxytocin also known as the love hormone, is disrupted. When your system is in threat or survival mode, your reproductive system goes offline, so to speak. The body mobilizes energy away from the internal organs, such as digestive and reproductive, and sends the energy to the extremities to increase capacity to fight or flee the situation.

Thus, the focus is on survival, not reproduction.

Another way of saying this is that when you are activated, your body is not in the position to digest food or reproduce. *Whoa.* I want to repeat this statement, because it is critical to understand: When the system is in survival mode or preservation mode, regardless if actual or perceived, the reproductive system goes offline. The focus is on survival, not reproduction.

The consequences of such an occurrence means that your physiology may have slowed down, stalled or shut down the progression of your labour. Further, your social bonding system, as discussed above, can become compromised. Thus, your body responds to environmental cues and attempts to keep you and your unborn baby safe.

From this perspective, your body is working for you during a stressful childbirth experience, not against you. The same goes for the postpartum period. Your social bonding system and the reproductive system come back online when, and only when, your body perceives its environment as safe again. Until then, the brain is stuck in hypervigilance and does not know that it is in fact 'safe' now.

Regardless of how much you may have tried to 'tell' yourself something different about the current situation, if your body is still in charge, it will not respond to the demands of your mind. Take the example of the mother who is challenged to bond with her newborn. Under a stressful circumstance, she may struggle to attune her attention to the newborn with open, connected, loving presence. And this often devastates the mother.

In a nutshell: Unresolved trauma makes it hard to feel alive and well in our body, mind, soul and relationships.

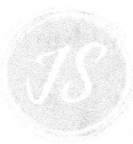

REFLECTIVE EXERCISE
ON TRAUMA

What does the statement *to disconnect from yourself* mean to you?

What happens when you are disconnected from yourself?

Why is it essential for you to remain connected to yourself?

Why is it important (and an integral part of healing) for you, as a parent, to remain connected to yourself?

What, where, and how do you access this core sense of self?

THERAPEUTIC ACTIVITY
VISUALIZATION EXERCISE

This activity encourages you to explore your feelings and thoughts associated with a new connection to your 'self'. You just learned a lot about the impact that trauma has on your core sense of self; resulting in feeling utterly disconnected. In this exercise, I invite you to consider the following.

As you think about reconnecting to this deeper aspect of yourself, and you consider the implications of remaining disconnected from this life force within, I invite you to image yourself as whole and fully alive. Note what this version of yourself looks like in the space below.

And now, I invite to feel the potential feelings associated with the whole version of yourself. Pay attention to the elevated emotions and hold the image with the elevated emotions for as long as you can. Pay attention to felt sensations in the body and notice any sensations being activated within the region of your heart. Hold it. Feel it. Fall in love with this image and version of yourself. Write about this experience in the space below.

CHAPTER 5

HOW BIRTH CAN INVOLVE TRAUMA

Why Do Mothers Commonly Experience Childbirth as Traumatic?

According to Peter Levine, a pioneering trauma theorist, childbirth is at risk of being potentially traumatizing for both mothers and baby. Childbirth is innately stressful and can be experienced as:
- Overwhelmingly painful.
- Risk or fear of death.
- Utter loss of control.
- A lack of power to avoid or escape situation.
- A sudden and/or shocking change in situation.
- A violating and/or abusive procedure.
- Isolating with a risk of abandonment.

All of these experiences can result in intense fear, panic and terror.

Current research on the outcomes of birth trauma:
- 1 out of 3 women are impacted by birth trauma.
- 2–7% of postpartum women will be diagnosed with postpartum post-traumatic stress disorder (P-PTSD).
- P-PTSD is reported as being under diagnosed (or misdiagnosed).
- Postpartum depression (PPD) affects 19%, or 1 out of 4, mothers.
- Postpartum anxiety (PPA) affects 16% of new mothers.
- Baby blues can affect up to 60–80% of new mothers.
- Childbirth trauma robs mothers' experiences of meaning.

- ★ The WHO has called for action and advocacy to eliminate disrespectful and abusive treatment in childbirth.
- ★ Trust in caregivers increases resiliency.
- ★ A mother's belief in the body's capacity to give birth increases resiliency.
- ★ Trauma-informed care is not mandated nor part of core curricula for many health professionals.

Giving birth is one of the most vulnerable experiences of a woman's life. If met with humiliation, violation, loss of control, and lack of capacity to protect her body, there is a high probability that a woman's stress system and threat response will become activated, thus initiating the body's threat instinct (fight/flight/freeze).

Women do not labour well under these conditions. In fact, they rarely give birth instinctively or without intervention when their stress response is activated. It is critical to note that childbirth is, in and of itself, a stressful event. However, what I am referring to is a toxic stress load (TSL) due to a perceived or real threat.

How Trauma Affects Others Involved

Not only can childbirth be traumatizing for the mother, but both the baby and any bystanders can suffer from similar trauma symptoms. It is important to note that witnessing a traumatic event, especially involving someone we love and where we feel utterly helpless and powerless, can be traumatic. As well, other medical professionals or support people, such as Doulas, Nurses, or partners, can also experience a flood of stress chemicals that leads to stored trauma.

However, when a support person 'checks out' it can be perceived by the woman in labour as a form of abandonment. The perception of 'checking out' or 'neglecting to respond' can later be used as a weapon between couples, creating friction and even more separation from each other and self.

I share this part because it is important to recognize that sometimes our behaviours are instinctual and not 'personal'. Thus, the disconnect you might have experienced during labour and delivery may not have been intended to cause harm or feel like neglect. Your partner or support people may have been unable to help you in the way they wanted to because they felt powerless to intervene and were experiencing a flood of stress hormones.

They too may need to reach out for support so that they can process the event and release emotions, thoughts and sensations that have remained stuck within their system. (For additional information, see the Resources section at the end of this guidebook.)

Identifying Stress and Trauma

Regardless of whether you feel your birth experience was traumatic or highly stressful, if you are still struggling to tell your birth story without emotional activation and if you're avoiding acknowledging or sharing the painful parts, it is very plausible that you have not fully integrated your birth experience.

I love the quote by Joe Dispenza that says, *"Wisdom is the result of trauma without the emotional charge."* There are most likely unresolved emotions, unresolved thoughts, and unresolved stress stored within your system that need your kind and compassionate attention so they can be released and restored. This is not wrong, nor does it indicate some failure on your part.

I like to remind my clients that a symptom—a distressing thought, emotion, felt sensation or memory—is offering information. These symptoms tell us something. They alone mean nothing until we label them with meaning. They are merely expressions and thus provide information about what in your system is unresolved. They are not wrong, nor bad.

If anything, your systems are telling you that something was very 'off' and disempowering about your birth experience. That you experienced an overwhelming amount of stress and that your system was sent into high gear in attempts to protect you and your baby. You went through a lot!

The fact that you are reading this book tells me that you have not sorted out the experience in your mind, body and heart. Something is still lingering and doesn't feel finished. And if you are similar to the hundreds of mothers I have worked with, you are likely carrying a narrative that sounds like: *What is wrong with me? Why can't I get over this? Will I be like this forever? Will I ever love my child? Am I a bad mom for feeling this way?*

A little reminder and pick-me-up:
Your body did not fail you.
You have done nothing wrong.
And your symptoms are not a sign of weakness.

Resiliency & Post-Traumatic Growth (PTG)

Innately, humans are resilient, and our systems can tolerate a fair amount of stress. In fact, stress is a necessary part of growth. For example, a newborn needs to experience stress throughout labour and birth because the chemicals associated with stress stimulate the nervous system and, at birth, trigger the babies instinct to breathe. This is healthy stress.

However, as you are learning, there is a tipping point for each one of us. This tipping point is unique and individual. So many factors impact our window of tolerance (as described above). That said, *post-traumatic growth*, a term coined by Martin Seligman and his research team, suggests that every time we integrate and restore our nervous system after a traumatic event we build resilience to tolerate stress.

The key is in the repair phase: how we repair, how quickly we repair, and how often we repair. It is like a muscle. Let's imagine that stress contracts the muscle fibres and can tear the fibres so that they grow bigger and stronger. Too much stress can rip the fibre and cause damage. We need to rest the muscle so that it can repair the damage. Eventually, the fibres strengthen and repair. If we provide a nourishing environment to help restore the muscle, we can trust that our biology will take care of the rest.

We need to offer the same kind of care and attention to help restore and repair the damages that our brain and heart have endured as a result of a trauma. It is not rocket science, however, for some reason when it comes to a 'brain injury'—mental unrest, including emotional disarray—humans respond in ways that are counter-intuitive, such as: resist, reject, punish, disconnect.

> **Therefore, supporting the notion that repair is a key ingredient in restoring the system back to health, we need to consider what is a nourishing response to a mother in the immediate postpartum.**

Further, it is encouraging to note that when you as a mother heal your nervous system and your heart after your difficult birth, you are also building resiliency and tolerance within the system of your newborn. You are influencing the health of your newborn simultaneously.

The following are resources and tools that can help you to integrate the experience and restore the nervous system after having experienced a traumatic childbirth. The focus is on repair, and highlighting strength of character and spirit.

Resources that support restoration of the nervous system:
- ★ Encouragement to talk about the event immediately following.
- ★ Care and support immediately following the event
- ★ Strong community and social connections.
- ★ Support by primary partner and caregivers.
- ★ Encouragement to find meaning (usually much later on).
- ★ Access to local resources.
- ★ Stress management skills.
- ★ Minimizing stressors (rest and limit visitors initially).
- ★ Loving relationships (love heals).
- ★ Yoga and movement.
- ★ Mindfulness and meditation.
- ★ Question your thoughts.
- ★ Get hormones checked.
- ★ Healthy nutrition (good fats and low sugars).
- ★ Nature.
- ★ Animals.

REFLECTIVE EXERCISE
ON CHILDBIRTH TRAUMA

Do you feel as if something was lost during childbirth? How about robbed or stolen? If yes, what was it?

Do you feel confused or disoriented by your birthing experience? What do you find most disorienting?

Do you sense that you are still back there, in your past experiences? If so, what are the loudest thoughts, feelings, sensations or images?

Are you trying to forget about it and just move on? How come?

Are you telling yourself that it wasn't that bad? Are you questioning why you're not 'over' it yet?

Deeper Reading

This bonus article, parts of which were originally printed in **Midwifery Today**, *takes a closer look at the impacts of childbirth stress during the post-partum period. I invite you to read this article to deepen your exploration and consolidate your learning to this point.*

How Childbirth-Related Stress May Be Contributing to Increased Postpartum Mood Disorders in New Mothers

Could the increased stress that mothers are experiencing before, during, and after childbirth be responsible for the rising rate of postpartum mood disorders?

This is a question I have asked myself countless time over the past 17 years as a student of Midwifery, Doula, childbirth educator and advocate, coach, maternal mental health researcher and more recently, a trauma-informed counsellor for mothers.

A woman's experience of pregnancy and childbirth is ever changing. How a woman experienced childbearing a century ago is vastly different than today. However, one thing has remained the same: It's a stressful life event. And, it's arguably more stressful now than it's ever been.

Mothers experience many kinds of stress throughout this precious period. The journey to motherhood is faced with challenges, which may present themselves during pregnancy, labour and birth, or the postpartum period. Childbirth is a time of great transition and change, and this change often includes arduous and challenging experiences. Yet, the mainstream mindset rarely endorses the idea that childbirth stressors are an important part of preparing for parenthood. As a result, rather than accept the challenges as part of a normal experience, many women are taught to resist the experience or approach it with fear.

Today, mothers are exposed to an enormous amount of information related to childbirth, as well as more medical testing during and after pregnancy. This is both a blessing and a curse. An increase in access to information is assumed to lead to increased safety and better birthing outcomes.

Yet, despite this, there's rising evidence that pregnancy is now a more stressful event for mothers than it's ever been. Rather than feeling empowered by information, many mothers are feeling overwhelmed by the number of decisions they need to make.

Pregnancy for the modern mother is met with a borage of testing, instructions, dos and don'ts, and decisions to be made about where to give birth, with whom, and how. This includes the constant hum of what if something goes wrong? In many cases, all of which creates new worries. In fact, many of the mothers I work with are equally worried about developing a postpartum mood disorder as they are about the birth itself. This is a notable change over the past decade.

What are the main stressors of the modern childbirth experience?

Let's pause for a moment to unpack the potential stressors experienced by mothers in today's world. Mothers are at risk of feeling stress from the moment they decide to try to conceive a baby or learn they are pregnant.

Stressors during pregnancy can include:
- Worries about miscarriage
- Worries about genetic dysfunction
- Worries about gestational diabetes
- Worries about developing pre-eclampsia
- Worries about risk associated with the Rh factor
- Worries about risks associated with Group B strep
- Concerns about nutrition; what to eat or what not to eat
- Concerns about environmental toxins
- Concerns about not receiving the caregiver you want
- Concerns about relationship challenges
- Changes in body
- Changes in role in the family
- Changes in work
- Increased financial stress and uncertainty about future funds
- Worries about the 'unknown' of parenthood
- Fear of not being able to give birth in the position you want
- Fear of not being in control during labor and birth
- Fear of childbirth pain
- Fear of interventions
- Fear of premature birth
- Fear of surgery
- Fear of having an unhealthy baby
- Fear of stillbirth
- Fear of dying during childbirth

In addition to these prenatal stressors, mothers also face labour and delivery stressors such as:

- Being overdue
- Waters breaking and not going into labour
- Needing an induction
- Labour being long and prolonged
- Feeling unsafe in labour
- Not knowing what is happening to the body during labour
- Feeling out of control in labour
- Feeling violated by procedures and protocols
- Not being able to make a choice in labour
- Bleeding during labour
- Not being able to tolerate the pain of contractions
- Needing an epidural in labour and being afraid of needles
- Not expecting what you are experiencing in labour
- Feeling observed and on display
- Not being listened to or not being able to voice needs
- Worrying about the wellbeing of baby
- Not understanding what symptoms mean
- Stalled labor
- Malposition of baby
- Lengthy pushing stage
- Being in an uncomfortable position and not being able to move
- Saying no or stop and not being listened to
- Needing an unplanned or emergency C-section
- Baby needing medical assistance during birth
- Mother losing a lot of blood after birth
- Mother having a difficult time delivering the placenta

And, to compound the stress of pregnancy, labour, and delivery, mothers often experience additional stressors in the postpartum period:

- Baby being sent to NICU immediately after birth
- Baby needing resuscitation after birth
- Mother and baby separated at birth (no skin to skin)
- Mother in recovery and baby with the other parent
- Mother having difficulty breastfeeding
- Mother lacking the instinct to bond with newborn
- Mother staying in hospital
- Mother being exhausted in the postpartum period
- Mother fighting with partner
- Mother feeling defeated by birth experience
- Mother lacking supports from friends, family, and caregivers
- Mother being told 'get over it'

Is it possible that these stressors are contributing to an increased risk of postpartum mood disorders for new mothers? Can you relate to any of these experiences? Is it postpartum mood disorders themselves that we should to be concerned with? Or, is the real concern the number of stressors that mothers experience in a short period of time?

French Obstetrician, Michel Odent, is well known for his strong opinions about supporting mothers' instinctive physiological needs during pregnancy and birth. His primary recommendation is for caregivers to do everything within their power to reduce unnecessary stress for the pregnant mother. The premise is that stress is the main reason for the challenges and complications that can arise throughout the childbearing continuum.

If an activated nervous system does not have the opportunity to return to homeostasis, it can remain in a state of hyper-arousal or hypo-arousal in which the system remains outside of what Dr. Dan Siegel calls the *window of tolerance*. The window of tolerance is the optimal zone of arousal in which our system can regulate and tolerate stressful information.

When a mother is **within the window of tolerance**, she can experience the following:
- Feel and think simultaneously
- Experience empathy
- Experience emotions as tolerable
- Demonstrate in-the-moment awareness
- Feel open and curious, rather than judgmental and defensive
- Awareness of boundaries (yours & others)
- Reactions adapt to fit the situation
- Feeling safe

When a mother is **outside of the window of tolerance**, she can experience the following as symptoms of **hyperarousal**:
- Tension or shaking
- Emotional reactivity
- Defensiveness
- Racing thoughts
- Intrusive imagery
- Emotional overwhelm
- Feeling unsafe
- Obsessive cognitive processing
- Hypervigilance
- Impulsivity
- Anger/rage

When a mother is **outside of the window of tolerance**, she can experience the following as symptoms of **hypoarousal**:

- ★ Numbing of emotions
- ★ No feelings
- ★ Disconnected
- ★ Ashamed
- ★ Reduced physical movement
- ★ Passive
- ★ Shut down/immobilized
- ★ Can't say no/reduced boundaries
- ★ Emotionally flat

When we remain within the window of tolerance, the social engagement system is activated and we can shift our attention towards others, including our newborns. When mothers are attuned and attached, mothers and newborn can relax into a state of calm, loving connection.

All of these are also important factors that reduce symptoms of postpartum mood disorders. Might it be wise to shift our focus towards reduction in childbirth-related stressors as a possible preventative measure for developing postpartum mood disorders?

I would argue that if we (as caregiver, family members, community members, and mothers) look for ways to reduce toxic stress load throughout the childbearing continuum, we may be able to significantly reduce the risk of mothers developing postpartum mood disorders.

Doing so would also increase the loving, calm connection circuitry (or, social bonding in love) that is innately wired in all humans. Evidence suggests that when a newborn experiences secure attachment during his or her primary period of development (during the first year), they are more likely to grow up with a healthy system—better immune function, better mental health, better physical health, better relational health, better sense of self.

This shift could be accomplished by looking at obstetrics, midwifery, and maternity care not only from a physical safety standpoint (reducing risk of maternal and infant mortality), but also from a neuro-physiological safety perspective (reducing risk by supporting the inner needs for emotional and mental safety).

In fact, I would argue that there needs to be a comprehensive paradigm shift in how we view birth. Currently, the medical mainstream mindset is that birth is a dangerous event and, therefore, needs to be managed through a medical lens.

Although it may be true, generally speaking, that childbirth is a physiologically stressful event, it does not need to be a psychologically stressful experience.

The body experiences stress naturally during pregnancy, labour, and birth. Although intended to help, modern approaches to obstetrics and midwifery can place additional external stressors on an already stressed mother. Much of this stress is linked to the perception of 'what if' something goes wrong, rather than actual life-threatening occurrences. This creates an accumulation of stress within the mother's nervous system and can trigger perceived harm or threat.

Until this shift occurs, there are some actions mothers can take to increase their window of tolerance, resulting in a greater degree of self-awareness, self-regulation, and compassion.

Simple actions that can increase a mother's window of tolerance:
- Practicing mindfulness and meditation
- Receiving support from others, especially from a partner that encourages, understands, listens, and loves
- Decreasing external stressors as much as possible, such as financial, relational, and environmental
- Engaging in imagery (visualization) exercises
- Journaling regularly
- Participating in creative activities, such as dancing, singing, poetry, writing, painting, pottery, or crafts
- Practicing yoga or other mindful-based physical activities
- Engaging in somatic experiencing or body-focused psychotherapy
- Participating with EMDR therapy
- Receiving binaural sound therapy and/or bi-lateral tapping
- Participating in relational psychotherapy
- Practicing breathing activities, such as progressive relaxation
- Contemplative practices to question stressful thoughts
- Being in nature
- Engaging in pet/equine therapy
- Talking about what you are experiencing with others
- Joining effective mother groups
- Developing and/or engaging in a spiritual practice

Postpartum mood disorders are complicated. They rarely appear as a stand-alone disorder. What causes a mother to experience symptoms of postpartum mood disorders is a multifaceted conversation. Each mother has a unique expression of past and present experiences that inform her nervous system, core beliefs, and sense of self.

Yet, when a mother experiences multiple, compounded stressful events during pregnancy, childbirth, and in the postpartum period, this stress is accumulated within her nervous system and, if left unresolved, can affect her overall mental health.

Since humans are resilient beings who innately thrive within secure and connected bonds of love, a larger emphasis on reducing stress and fostering love towards the self and others, could be a powerful way to avoid the symptoms of postpartum mood disorders in new mothers.

CHAPTER 6

MAKING SENSE OF YOUR GRIEF

Grief as Medicine

Last chapter you learned about trauma and how it impacts the whole person: brain health, relationship health, physical health, spiritual health, and mental health. Mostly, how trauma disconnects you from your core self.

You may or may not have identified your childbirth experience with the term 'birth trauma', however, if you are reading this guidebook, you likely have unprocessed and unexpressed grief about your childbirth experience. This includes any stressful event throughout the entire continuum from conception to immediate postpartum.

According to Jane Simington, you can have grief without trauma, but you cannot have trauma without grief[8]. When there is unresolved grief stored within your heart, resolution and healing cannot occur. Let's take a deeper look at how a mother can be impacted by unexpressed, unacknowledged, and unprocessed grief. *(Note: A portion of this section was originally published on the MCAN website as a guest post.)*

Expressing Grief

What is disenfranchised grief? A traumatic childbirth experience, at any point throughout the continuum of childbirth, that resulted in an unexpected birth outcome can trigger a type of grief that is called disenfranchised grief.

---
8   *Simington, Trauma Recovery Certification Handbook.*

> **Disenfranchised grief** is a type of grief expressed that is
> not recognized, nor honoured, by the dominant culture.

A birth that resulted in a *loss of a dream birth vision* is rarely acknowledged by others as a legitimate form of grief. And yet, grief is an instinctive emotional reaction to having lost something of deep importance—relationship, identity, environment, finances, health.

There is also a form of deep grief that can arise during transitional turning points in life that have gone unacknowledged. Let's call this *life cycle grief*; it is linked to *our lack of honouring 'rites of passage'*.

During a rite of passage, traditionally, people would be initiated into a new phase of life, a new purposeful being. The initiate would be confronted with an arduous experience that they would find their way through by calling on their inner strengths. In the process, they shed old parts of themselves to embrace the new emerging self. The intensity of the event was intended to induce pain and discomfort so the person would 'let go' and grieve the 'undoing of what was'.

We no longer encourage rites of passage in our dominant culture and we discourage grieving when a part of our old self has gone through something arduous. This creates a dilemma.

How can you claim yourself as a mother if you have not been honoured the chance to grieve your old self and old life? (Never mind the fact that you also need to grieve the losses you experienced throughout your childbirth experience.)

When we think about grief, we usually think of it as a response to death. And yet, there are many different kinds of losses that we can and need to grieve such as:

- ★ Identity loss.
- ★ Environmental loss.
- ★ Relationship loss/divorce/relocation.
- ★ Loss of health.
- ★ Loss of hopes and dreams.
- ★ Death of a loved one.
- ★ Death of pets.
- ★ Loss of job (financial insecurity).

Childbirth is a time in a woman's life where she is shedding her old self, her securities and her past way of life to make room for this new phase and stage of her life called motherhood. The lack of support, encouragement and ceremony surrounding the initiation of childbirth is often met with a sense of incompleteness, hollowness and confusion. All of this, layered by the complications of having experienced a traumatic childbirth, can send any mother into a real tizzy.

Let's take a look at the impact of ignoring to honour this very precious time, the postpartum.

Grief and Isolation in the Postpartum

There is a rising dilemma experienced by many mothers during the postpartum, including years after birth, which is rarely discussed within the childbirth communities, academic journals, or amongst birth professionals. Sure, it may be referenced a few times here and there, and yes, there is public acknowledgment of the terms 'disempowered childbirth' or 'traumatic birth', but what are the consequences of such occurrences?

The predicament I am referring to is the effects of disenfranchised grief and social isolation due to unplanned childbirth interventions that contributed to an unexpected negative or traumatic childbirth experience. Let's unpack the concept of both of those terms, the consequences of such, and how we (mothers and community members) can attempt to address this problem.

It is important to note that *the event itself* (what actually happened during the pregnancy, birth, and postpartum) and *the individual perception of the event* are both contributing factors that influence how well a mother integrates, makes sense of, and resolves what happened during her childbirth experience.

Two mothers could experience a similar unfolding of events and each of their perceptions of that experience will be different, which means that the impact of the experience will be stored differently within their nervous system and brain. How we perceive an event is influenced by many factors such as and not limited to: past events, family and childhood experiences, beliefs, current events, cultural and community beliefs, capacity for dual awareness, state of wellbeing, dominant worldview, amount of oppression and marginalization, and overall mental health before the event occurred.

Thus, the impact of a mother's childbirth experience is unique with a dynamic interplay of both internal and external influences. All of which influences how she thinks, feels, and responds in the postpartum.

Research suggests that the quicker a mother can process and integrate what has occurred, the less likely she will present with symptoms of postpartum mood disorders[9]. One of the ways mothers integrate highly charged emotional information is through *expressed grief*.

Grief is a state experience that airs itself in response to a loss or death. It encompasses a multitude of emotions and includes non-linear stages of expression such as: denial, anger, shock, guilt, shame, sadness, confusion, blame.

---

[9] Grekin and O'Hara, "Prevalence and Risk Factors of Postpartum Post-traumatic Stress Disorder: A Meta-Analysis"; Sarah R Edwards, Lindsey Devries, and Aleska R Hagan, "Risk Factors for Postpartum PTSD : Coercion During Labor and History of Abuse," 2014, 10-11.

As we already discussed, disenfranchised grief is a type of unacknowledged grief that occurs when culture, family, and community lack understanding and support towards the aired grief[10]. In such conditions a mother feels alone and confused by her emotions when those who matter the most to her, and society at large, do not grant permission to grieve. Most likely, it is not that those around her do not support her grief, but rather they lack understanding or do not know *how* to offer support.

Hence, the grief becomes internalized and suppressed, and an internal negative dialogue takes over intensifying an already challenging situation. One can imagine that if a mother has unexpressed grief along with a negative mindset about herself and her birth experience, the likelihood of having difficulty in the postpartum increases, followed by a growing probability of being diagnosed with a postpartum mood disorder.

What presents is unexpressed grief and internalized emotional and mental pain that was accumulated by the high degree of physiological stress throughout the childbirth continuum, resulting in no outlet to restore 'self' back to homeostasis—a balanced state of wellbeing.

What was lost?

Mothers who had unplanned, unwanted or unexpected medical interventions at any point throughout the continuum of childbirth can experience the following losses: loss of birth dream and vision; loss of physical health; disconnection to self; loss of financial stability; loss of career or vocation; loss of relationships; loss of spiritual connection; loss of mental faculty.

One can imagine the energetic outpouring and attachment that occurs when a mother spends nine months or more imagining, dreaming, learning, anticipating, and planning for a certain kind of childbirth experience. To then be met with a completely different and unexpected occurrence than what was planned or envisioned...

> It is thus normal to experience disappointment and grief when that expected event turns out to be a different reality than initially planned.

Attached to a mother's childbirth experience are all of the thoughts, feelings, smells, sensations, and images that produced an emotional response. Thus, the event is encoded with all of this information causing neurons to fire together, and thus wire together, cultivating what neuroscientists call 'a neural network' of

---

10   *Simington, Trauma Recovery Certification Handbook.*

associated information[11]. If this information was processed as stressful, terrifying, disempowering, painful etc. the memory will be stored as such.

Within the continuum of childbirth, the stress response could be triggered due to the following: feeling out of control; lacking informed consent and choice; aggressive or unwanted physical exams; violating procedures; strangers as caregivers; intrusive sounds, lights, people; overwhelming pain; terror of harm for baby and/or self.

Distress, disappointment, and sadness are valid responses to such an experience. A mother who experienced something similar needs the space and encouragement to be allowed to cry, share, express anger and guilt, and come to terms with what happened. And yet, I have witnessed mothers quickly attempt to cover up those feelings of distress.

For many they experience shame in expressing their grief. There is a sense that *'it is not okay to feel sad because my baby is healthy.'* This sentiment furthers the gap of isolation.

Mothers cannot heal in isolation.

When a mother is negatively impacted by her childbirth experience, has unexpressed grief, and lacks support to process and integrate the event, her risk of being isolated in her emotions, thoughts, and sensations can escalate. As social beings, we heal in relationship to one another[12]. This lack of belonging comes as a surprise to many of the mothers I work with.

Allow me to elaborate. Let's look at the scenario of a mother who was planning to have a natural childbirth that resulted in an unplanned Caesarean birth. Prior to her perceived negative childbirth experience this mother was a part of the natural childbirth community. She joined a natural birthing class, attended a yoga or pregnancy movement class, joined online forums and blogs, talked with other mothers who gave birth naturally, and had a prenatal cohort. During pregnancy there was a sense of *belonging*—to something meaningful and purposeful.

However, the secondary loss of no longer belonging to a 'community' of mothers who can relate to one another has added another layer of grief to an already complicated situation.

---

11 Siegel, "Toward an Interpersonal Neurobiology of the Developing Mind: Attachment Relationships, 'Mindsight,' and Neural Integration"; Siegel, Mindsight: The New Science of Personal Transformation; Dispenza, Breaking the Habit of Being Yourself: How to Lose Your Mind and Create a New One.

12 Badenoch, Being a Brain Wise Therapist: A Practical Guide To Interpersonal Neurobiology; Shari M Geller and Stephen W Porges, "Therapeutic Presence: Neurophysiological Mechanisms Mediating Feeling Safe in Therapeutic Relationships," Journal of Psychotherapy Integration, 2014, doi:10.1037/a0037511; Stephen W. Porges, "The Polyvagal Theory: New Insights into Adaptive Reactions of the Autonomic Nervous System," Cleveland Clinic Journal of Medicine 76, no. SUPPL.2 (2009): 86–90, doi:10.3949/ccjm.76.s2.17.

And in my experience, these mothers are sitting in silence with their grief, unsure how to integrate what has happened, and questioning where and if they belong to any group.

To understand more clearly what I mean by different childbirth 'groups', I believe it is essential to distill what I call the different camps of childbirth:

Camp A: Natural physiological childbirth
Camp B: Planned, medically-assisted childbirth
Camp C: Unplanned, medically-intervened childbirth

Natural (Camp A) vs. medical (Camp B) childbirth has been in opposition for years now, since the introduction of medical interventions and OB/GYNs. Rarely do these camps see eye-to-eye, although they have seen a growing tolerance for one other.

For nearly the past two decades, I can honestly say that there is still a strong *Us vs. Them* mentality when it comes to the midwifery model of care versus the medical model of care. (For those who want to read more about this, Robbie Davis-Floyd, a medical and cultural anthropologist, offers lots of insightful discourse on this topic.)

Fundamentally, each model of care has differing points of view. This is not about which model is better, but rather, let's acknowledge that they are different. And what I am noticing surface is a third contingent of mothers who perceive that they no longer ascribe themselves to either model.

These are the silenced voices of mothers who aligned with the natural birthing community and had a childbirth experience that resulted in an unplanned and most often, *unwanted medically assisted* (intervened) birth.

These mothers make up the majority of those who are coming forward to process their grief and trauma associated with their childbirth experience. Until recently, these mothers did not have a 'term' to describe what they are experiencing. They have been silenced due to internalized shame, confusion, disconnection, and externalized expectations.

The Current Problem
It is silently agreed upon and tolerated that Camp A, natural physiological childbirth, and Camp B, planned, medically-assisted childbirth, have differing opinions, and often when mothers get together they *choose* to not discuss their differing perspectives and choices of childbirth.

Many mothers feel supported within a community of mothers with like-minded parenting and birthing worldviews, and they rarely venture outside of this cohort. Thus, they are not isolated and they belong. However, mothers from Camp C experience something different—they belong to neither Camp A nor Camp B. They are often afraid to speak about the event, especially if they are grateful for the medical support they received. Rarely do they have space to speak authentically about what happened and how they feel, nor do they feel safe to process their grief.

I have heard numerous mothers say that they refrain from sharing their birth experiences because they do not want to sound like they are complaining or negatively impacting another mother's perception of childbirth. Often, these mothers internalize their grief as being a sign of weakness.

This lack of belonging, which contributes to the psychological and social isolation I spoke about earlier, can hinder the healing process for such a mother. Given that humans are social beings[13] the psychological impact of social isolation within the postpartum can be far-reaching. As a therapist, I've observed **a common theme amongst mothers who have experienced their birth to be both disempowering and traumatic: loneliness.**

The following is a list of observed attributes of loneliness:
- ★ Mothers don't want to be around other mothers who had positive birthing experiences because they are afraid of being judged for 'not doing it right'.
- ★ Mothers don't want to hear about other positive births because it is too painful.
- ★ Mothers don't want to share about their birth for fear of making other pregnant women afraid of childbirth.
- ★ Mothers are angry, but do not feel justified in their anger.
- ★ Mothers are grieving but feel confused about their grief.
- ★ Mothers feel that their body failed them or that they did something wrong.
- ★ Mothers stop going to mothering groups because they feel they can no longer relate.
- ★ Mothers rarely tell other mothers that they are in therapy.
- ★ Mothers don't feel supported by their primary partner or family members.
- ★ Mothers hide their deeper truth.
- ★ Mothers feel childbirth has changed them and they no longer relate to their old way of thinking but are afraid to comment on this.

---

13 Badenoch, *Being a Brain Wise Therapist: A Practical Guide To Interpersonal Neurobiology*; Porges, "Love: An Emergent Property of the Mammalian Autonomic Nervous System"; Porges, "The Polyvagal Theory: New Insights into Adaptive Reactions of the Autonomic Nervous System," 2009.

A Proposed New Role

Although many mothers feel silenced or isolated in their experiences, there is an emerging voice that is beginning to surface. My hope is that these mothers can offer encouragement and support to others.

This group of sprouting mothers who are reaching out for support and courageously choosing to heal (like you!) **have an important role and influence within the childbirth community**—*they are bridging between two worldviews.*

Let's take a closer look at this notion.

What is a bridge person?
A bridge person is someone who can close the gap between one point of view and another point of view because they can offer insight and perspective based upon experience.

This new role cultivates meaning and fosters a new sense of belonging amongst mothers and families. These brave voices will hopefully help to eliminate the *Us vs. Them* mentality that overtly or subtly positions mothers against one another. We need more connection as mothers, and less shaming or shunning for childbirth choices.

How can you become a bridge person?
To begin, there is a need to **own one's story** and begin to share it, even if the story is unfinished and contains sadness, anger, frustration. There are many stories of birth. We need to hear *all* stories of birth, each unique tale, and engage with curiosity.

Your story is *as* important as every other birth story told. It offers a different perspective on birth. For some mothers, birth is hard, surprising, challenging, scary, confusing, disempowering, isolating and unexpected. And yet, even in all of that, there is still power, understanding, opportunity to heal, insight, transformation and an experience that brings mothers to their edge.

There is no right or wrong way to give birth. There are many ways to experience childbirth. Together, we can begin to heal. Sometimes to be fully received with open presence by other mothers and family members is enough to start your healing process. Simply **knowing that your experience *is as valid* as everyone else's is a powerful form of healing.** When humans are truly received, we feel like we matter and we belong. Belonging is one of our deepest innate drives.

We need each other, bottom line. And, for some, belonging and being heard can help to shift unprocessed emotions about a negative childbirth experience towards deeper understanding and acceptance. Therefore, it is critical that we work towards inclusion so that mothers can rise strong together.

REFLECTIVE EXERCISE
ON GRIEF

When I think about my childbirth experience, I am grieving the loss(es) of:

How has my grief not been honoured by society?

What scares me most about expressing my grief?

What does 'expressing my grief' mean to me? What does it look like?

What do I need so that I can safely express my grief?

CHAPTER 7

Letting Go of Blame and Anger

The Culture of Blame

Before we engage directly with the topic of anger, let's take a moment and explore the concept of blame and how it shows up in the arena of birth. We are living in an epidemic of what I call *blame culture*. I want to talk about how the natural birth ideology is at times a contributing factor to the rise in childbirth shame and blame.

As a pioneer of the natural birth industry, of which includes a strong focus on instinctive and physiological labour and birth, I held a strong motivation to teach about the power of birth through the lens of undisturbed birth. All of which was supported by scientific evidence in the fields of physiology, endocrinology, neuroscience, personal experience and a belief that the mammalian female body was designed to give birth instinctively.

I became a spokesperson for natural birth after the birth of my first child because I saw birth as a women's rights issue; I wanted to stop violence against women in birth. Naturally, I saw the medical institution as the culprit (and those who worked within it) and midwifery as the solution.

I believe that all passion is motivated initially from a place of heart and soul; a desire to 'do good' and 'help'. However, while the initial motivation stemmed from a place to 'do no harm', it is hard to maintain that place of pure motivation without developing an ideology.

Fifteen years deep into the world of birth, I was still grappling with the question: If birth is physiological and instinctive than why is it not the experience for so many labouring mothers? What stands in the way of accessing this mammalian birth right? And why does it matter?

For years I believed that if caregivers would just support birth physiology and get out of the way with all of their protocols and interventions, then women would birth instinctively and uncomplicated most of the time. This led to a belief that the reason why there is a high rate of complicated births, followed by unwanted C-sections and interventions, was/is the caregivers' 'fault' for not supporting a mother's physiology and neglecting to apply evidence-based care.

From this vantage point the 'cure' was/is simple (or so I thought): Caregivers need to change their practices to be supportive of physiological and instinctive birth.

The First Layer of Blame
This mindset led towards what I would consider to be the first layer of blame: If childbirth did not turn out the way the mother had hoped, someone is to be blamed, and that someone was the caregiver.

For a few years I was stuck in this mindset and could not see beyond it: *Caregivers of birth (OB/GYN, midwives, nurses) were at fault, the system was at fault, and the education was at fault.* Mothers could scapegoat their painful feelings by adopting this mindset. Instead of authentic grief being expressed in response to their unwanted birthing experience, mothers could project anger towards the institution of birth and make them 'wrong'.

This anger has fueled many movements within childbirth:
- ★ Freebirth/unassisted birthing.
- ★ Cesarean prevention and awareness.
- ★ Mainstreaming midwifery.
- ★ Childbirth rights.
- ★ Thousands of blogs and videos.
- ★ Documentaries about the politics in childbirth.
- ★ Lawsuits against mistreatment in labour.

These movements have opened up a conversation that giving birth is no longer a private affair, but rather a public topic of conversation.

Within nearly two decades I have personally witnessed the business of birth BOOM! A doula is no longer a puzzling-sounding word with no context, but rather a necessity for pregnant families to have by their side. In fact, we have experienced an explosion within the doula industry. There are more courses and instructors now, more doulas, more online programs, extra workshops and birth bag supplies to be purchased, and more postpartum doulas.

When you are pregnant, you are bombarded with more than a handful of different childbirth classes to take, all of which are most often focused on helping you have a 'natural' childbirth experience. Some even focus on hypnotherapy to help you train your brain to 'let go' in labour so you can have a pain-free physiological labour.

Midwifery has become mainstream (for the most part) and more and more people are hearing the word and choosing a midwife as their primary caregiver. For pregnant families within my home city of Edmonton, many are being denied access to care because there are not enough midwives to serve the demand. Met with outraged citizens, many of these women who are denied access of care are afraid to give birth with an OB/GYN in attendance. (I was one of these women who feared care from an OB/GYN.)

The Second Layer of Blame
This feeds what I call the second layer of blame: that the system has denied women access to a caregiver of choice and it is therefore the system's fault for an unwanted birth outcome.

Again, outrage in regard to 'lack of choice' has motivated a movement to draw awareness to the fact that this lack of choice is a violation of birth rights. This has led to what I would call the second wave of unassisted birthers. The first wave was motivated by a desire to have autonomy and ownership over the birth experience, while the second wave is in response to a denial of care. Two different starting points, but a similar ending point.

In all of this, the natural birth movement is still very much at the forefront of the waves. From what I have gathered over the years, more women are desiring a natural birth because of a belief that this is the best way to give birth. And although part of me believes that this is true, I cannot know that it is the absolute truth— especially if it is causing much emotional pain amongst today's mothers. Birth empowerment and informed choice are high up on the needs list for pregnant women.

In the past, I taught exactly this: if you just get the right caregiver (or no caregiver), who supports birth physiology and altered states, and who listens to you and supports your needs, you will feel safe enough to let birth happen to you.

I felt women needed the right environment to support their hormonal needs in labour. I believed women needed to be undisturbed and left alone so they could find their way. Yet, I still found myself perplexed when I attended a birth like this that 'didn't work out'.

What went wrong?
Who interrupted the labour?
Who was to blame?

Underneath these initial responses were thoughts that something got in the way: It must have been due to hidden unprocessed trauma, discomfort with letting go, psychological challenges, unhappy relationships, discomfort with sexuality, discomfort with losing control, low pain tolerance, an unsupportive environment, and so on.

As you can see, there are thousands of possibilities, some of which may have contributed to the outcome, many of which may not have. Now, rather than focus on 'figuring it out', I've learned that a more important question is: **Was the mother supported in a kind, considerate, dignified way as she gave birth?**

The Third Layer of Blame
This leads to a third layer of blame: I, the mother, must be at fault. My body failed me because I didn't have the outcome I wanted—the outcome that society is suggesting I have. Anything less is unforgivable, and someone needs to be blamed.

WHEN THERE IS BLAME, THERE IS SHAME.

Each of these three layers of blame fosters shame and, worse, distrust in yourself (including your body for future births) and others (e.g. caregivers). This cultivates the very thing that I, as an advocate of natural birth, was trying to eradicate from the very beginning: violence against women in childbirth. I can't believe it has taken me this long to realize this and see through the cracks.

What is worse: externalized violence or internalized self-perpetuated violence?
Violence is violence and they both feed disempowerment and oppression. Internalized shame is a violent act that disempowers every mother, diminishes her life force, keeps her from feeling joy with her children, feeds the belief that the female body is defective, and separates mothers from each other.

Instead, we need to foster a society that **empowers** mothers and families. I am honoured to hold mothers' stories of shame and guilt as I sit on the receiving end and see the damage that can be caused by a birth ideology that sounds like: *all women must give birth physiologically, naturally, and instinctively.*

I am humbled as I sit in sessions and hold raw grief—grief that is behind the anger and the blame, and grief that comes from relief and release from these binding mindsets: **grief that happens when a mother realizes she doesn't have to hold onto the blame.** Mothers are encouraged to focus on discovering a new mindset that fosters kindness towards self and other. From this kind inner place, true joy can flourish regardless of one's birth experience.

Note: I am not suggesting that we turn a blind eye and ignore overt abuse that does occur in childbirth. This type of childbirth trauma needs addressing and consequences. There is no room for violence. Period.

REFLECTIVE EXERCISE
ON ANGER AND BLAME

"Holding on to anger is like grasping a hot coal with the intent of throwing it at someone else; you are the one who gets burned" ~ The Buddha

What do you usually do with your anger? *When I am angry I usually...*

How is that behaviour serving you or your family? Would you like to let it go?

Growing up, what were you told you could or could not do with anger?

What was lost, stolen, taken, fractured, or injured during your birth experience?

During your birth experience, which of your needs were not met?

What do you wish you had voiced, but could not, because you were frozen or too afraid?

What thoughts or judgments do you have towards feeling angry about your birth experience?

How does anger fuel you? What do you 'get' from being angry?

THERAPEUTIC ACTIVITY
NARRATIVE EXERCISE

This activity encourages you to explore residual anger and blame. **Who are you holding accountable for your experience; who do you want to punish?** We cannot completely integrate and resolve in our hearts and minds what happened when we are holding onto anger and blame.

We live in a culture that seeks to 'blame' and 'punish' as a means to find resolution. However, in the restorative justice model for healing, the wronged person or community does not seek to punish with shame. Rather, the intent is to open up dialogue to encourage true regret to surface. In this space, hearts open and each member acknowledges the humanity of each person.

When there is trauma there is pain, and often we *want* to hold someone or something accountable. Although it may be appropriate to hold someone or something accountable, we need to ask the question: **How long do I want to hold onto this anger and blame? Who is it serving? How is it serving?**

Anger has purpose and is an important part of trauma resolution and recovery. In the wild, mammals roar and rage to complete the trauma response and restore the nervous system back to homeostasis. Raging can 'move it out of the system' and running like a wild animal releases the pent-up energetic charge cultivated by an activated stress response.

However, humans are rarely encouraged to experience their anger. Anger is labeled as scary, bad, harmful, hurtful. Thus, we are left to negotiate our anger internally, which can complicate our healing. Holding on to the anger and suppressing it causes more harm. It needs to be discharged from the body in a safe way.

I encourage you to reflect upon the following notion and **allow felt sensations to arise within your body.** When you feel ready, begin to write using the spaces that follow.

When I think about my childbirth experience, I blame the following people because...

If you blamed yourself or your body, write down what you are feeling. *I am feeling...*

If you blamed a caregiver, someone else, or something else, write down who you blamed and how you feel:

Take a moment to **notice your internal dialogue** (your thoughts) and pay attention to the tone, voice, language and words that came out.

Write down all of your stressful and judgmental thoughts. **This is your internal narrative.** These are the 'stories' you are telling yourself about the situation. *(For example: My body failed me. I wish I had done something different. They neglected me and should have monitored things more closely. They were incompetent. They violated me. I wish I would have said something. Why didn't I speak up?)*

Now let's go deeper.

Explore the statements above. **Pay attention to one or two thoughts that really bother you.** Which thoughts generate a large amount of distress?

Notice if you are trying to stay distant from the felt sensations or if you are trying to reason with yourself and lessen the impact of the thought itself. We often try to reason with our thoughts to minimize the impact they are having on us.

Now that you have determined the two thoughts that are most uncomfortable for you to consider or believe, write them down below.

Stressful thought one:

Stressful thought two:

Usually what we are most uncomfortable with are the hidden messages or beliefs that are 'behind' or underneath the original stressful thought.
To access this belief, we must go deeper and ask the question:
When I believe this thought, it is upsetting to me because...

What am I telling **MYSELF** about **MYSELF** in this situation?
I am telling myself...

Cheat sheet time! Some of these internalized core beliefs sound like the following:

I am bad	*I am weak*
I am wrong	*I am powerless*
I am inadequate	*I am disgusting*
I am a failure	*I am alone*
I did something wrong	*I am unsafe*
I am unworthy	*I am insignificant*
I am unlovable	*I am hopeless*

When you have completed this exercise:
Grab a small hand towel and roll it up tightly, and squeeze it with force. Notice body sensations and allow the sensation associated with anger to build internally. Start twisting the towel tightly and keep twisting until all the energy has moved throughout your body.

You may feel tingling sensations, you may want to make noise, you may feel like crying, you may feel like shaking and you may feel exhausted. Just notice all those sensations and follow your instinct as it arises to release this energy.

The energy of anger will not last long if you **let it move through you and out of you.** Let the towel absorb the energy of anger. Keep breathing and stay with your breath throughout. This is a simple and effective way to move anger. It's an exercise you can also teach to your child(ren).

When you feel like you have released the energy, or part of the energy, ask yourself the following: **What would I like to BELIEVE about MYSELF in regard to my childbirth experience?**

I did…

I am…

I will…

Even if you do not believe this new perspective yet, you are starting to hold the potential for this new possibility within your mind's eye. Notice if you have any new feelings or emotions that surface with this new potential belief. Are those feelings different? How do they differ? I am not asking that you believe the new thought—just hold the potential and feel what it would be like if you could embrace this new thought.

For example:

I did the best I could.
I will get better.
I am enough.
I am okay as I am.
I am safe now.

We are just beginning to prime your mind to hold the potential that you will think and feel differently about your birth experience. But for now, it is important to access the limiting beliefs that are acting like the gatekeepers between 'how you want to think and feel' and 'how you are actually thinking and feeling'. We will explore more of the 'mindset' stuff in the Chapter Seven on perception.

> **Note:** Remember that you are in charge of this exercise and process. If at any time it doesn't feel right to you, or you are feeling too much, listen to those instincts and stop. Take a breath and use one of your calming techniques. If you sense that you need professional support to help guide you through this process and discharge the emotional energy from your system, jump to the resource list on my website for additional support.

CHAPTER 8

Learning to Trust Your Body Again

Childbirth Physiology 101

Let's start with some concepts to consider about your childbirth that you may not have been taught or told:

* Your body was working for you, not against you.
* Your body did not fail you.
* Oxytocin is compromised when adrenaline is in the system.
* You are a mammal with instincts and a prefrontal cortex that often gets in the way of birth.
* Birth does not unfold instinctively in 'normal' beta-brain wave reality. Rather, we give birth from an altered state of consciousness.
* Childbirth professionals are not trained to protect your neuro-physiological needs for childbirth. Rather, they are trained to protect you and your baby from dying at all costs.
* If you were stuck in a fear response, it would have been very challenging to birth physiologically without medical management of labour. *This does not mean you did something wrong or that your body failed you.*
* Birth is an extension of your sexual health and your sexual life.

Let's take a moment and unpack each of these statements.

Your body was working for you, not against you; your body did not fail you.
This is a loaded statement in and of itself. Almost every mother I have spoken with who feels devastated by her birth experience believes that her body failed her.

This belief that "I did something wrong" is based in an old imprint that has been fostered by a dominant worldview that keeps you feeling small. It blames you and it feeds guilt and shame. We know that we do not heal from these places.

Although it may feel real and true that your body failed you, I am proposing something utterly different here. I'm proposing that regardless of what happened and why it happened, your body did not fail you. It was working for you, not against you.

Whoa. "How is this possible?" you might ask. If you were told by your care provider that your body failed to progress, or your baby got stuck because your passage was too small, this might sound surprising.

It is actually quite simple, and physiology does not lie. Most likely your nervous system reacted to either your external environment or your internal environment (your perceptions). Your reaction was possibly one of fear and stress, activating your survival response and causing your system to become dysregulated.

Thus, feeling way too much. Followed by a perception that you cannot do anything about it, resulting in disharmony within your mind, body and heart. Dysregulation interrupts your flow of natural birthing hormones (see below) and causes you to fight against your instinctive stress response. If you're unable to resolve your stress response, by discharging the energy, you may have remained in a state of high alert during your whole labour, with intent of protecting yourself and your baby.

Your body was actually trying to protect you, not cause complications.

And so, this contributes and results in the next statement...

If you were stuck in a threat response, it would have been very challenging to birth physiologically without medical management of labour, and
this does not mean you did something wrong or that your body failed you.
Just that. Your body did not fail you. It was responding instinctively.

Oxytocin is compromised when adrenaline is in the system

> *'The parallels between making love and giving birth are clear, not only in terms of passion and love, but also because we need essentially the same conditions for both experiences: privacy and safety."*
> ~ Dr. Sarah J Buckley, author of 'Gentle Birth, Gentle Mothering'

Let's explore the hormonal blueprint of labour and birth as outlined in Sarah Buckley's latest research[14]. The following are the hormones that are necessary and present throughout a physiological labour and delivery.

1. **Oxytocin** contracts smooth soft tissues (uterus) and is responsible for instigating the instinct to bond. It is also considered to be the love hormone. Oxytocin initiates labour and is released throughout as well as at the peak moment of birth, while breastfeeding, during touch, orgasm, and death.
2. **Endorphins**, known as the pleasure hormone, are the body's natural pain relief. They are released throughout labour.
3. **Catecholamines** are part of the adrenaline family and are responsible for exciting the system and energizing for mobility. Catecholamines are released as baby is being born.
4. **Prolactin** is considered to be the mothering hormone and is responsible for breastmilk production.

What is the optimal environment that supports the optimal flow of these birthing hormones?

Many natural childbirth experts have written about the optimal environment for labour and delivery. The main consensus is that a woman in labour must feel safe and secure, primarily.

The following is a brief list that supports the neurobiological needs of a woman in labour. The following needs are recommended:

⋆ A need for safety and security.
⋆ A need for calm presence both from others and from the self.
⋆ A need to feel connected to loved ones.
⋆ A need for privacy and darkness.
⋆ A need for warmth to support the flow of hormones.
⋆ A need for trust in the process from both others and the self.
⋆ Caregivers who offer loving kind support.
⋆ A need to feel in control of surroundings and choices.
⋆ A need to consent.

Stop for a moment and consider: were any of these needs *not* met during your childbirth experience? If so, which ones?

---

14 Buckley, "Hormonal Physiology of Childbearing: Evidence and Implications for Women, Babies, and Maternity Care."

Let's explore the notion of safety a bit further.

Both internal and external environmental stressors must be minimized to support the altered state experience of childbirth. We could argue that external safety is beyond our control—sometimes this is true. However, generally speaking, women in labour seem to believe that their external environment is 'safe', regardless of where they choose to give birth.

However, if at any moment throughout the labour process the mother *perceived* that her external environment was no longer safe—that a person or thing was threatening or unpredictable—this would have activated her stress response. Further, pain can be perceived as unsafe, triggering the threat response and encoding in the brain that contractions are 'dangerous'. This gives rise to an example of how both the external or internal environment can be perceived as 'unsafe'.

You are a mammal with instincts and a prefrontal cortex that often gets in the way of birth, because birth does not unfold instinctively in 'normal' beta brain reality. Rather, we give birth from an altered state of consciousness.
Now that is a mouthful. What are beta brain wave states? And what exactly does altered state of consciousness mean?

When we are in a normal everyday rational thinking state, we are in a brain wave state called 'beta'. There are different levels of beta waves and high beta, indicates survival state. Beta has a frequency associated with it, and that frequency is linked to linear thinking, problem solving, conversational, focused, and astute attention. This also correlates with the functions of our left hemisphere of the brain.

Although we love engaging with our left hemisphere because it gives us a sense of being in control, in contrast, we labour and birth through engagement with the right hemisphere. The right hemisphere is associated with non-linear experiences, creativity, expansiveness, spontaneity and flow. As such, when we are in these states, our brain wave patterns change. The frequency of energy and information slows down. There are a few different slower frequencies that are measured as being associated with different states of consciousness: alpha, theta, and delta. Gamma is a super state, in which mystical and ecstatic experiences present.

Alpha is known as the bridge frequency that carries us into theta. Alpha is experienced as the 'day dreaming' state. When we are in alpha we feel relaxed, present and often in states of imagination or visualization. Creativity flows from alpha and a doorway to the sub-conscious is opened.

Theta is considered to be the 'healing state'. You may have heard of *theta healing* before (if not, Google it!). When we are in this state of openness, receptivity, and deep relaxation, we can access deeper knowledge and intuition.

The practice of meditation moves us into this state, and it can be experienced as a warm sensation and a calm comfort.

Delta is the deep abyss, the deep waters of the unconscious. We are usually not aware of being in delta. Our sense of self and body disappear in this state. However, brain scans can pick up this state and those in delta are very aware and conscious. When we sleep, we move through all of these brain wave states.

There is one more brain wave state called **gamma**. Gamma is akin to ecstasy. Gamma is a high frequency brain wave state that is associated with mystical experiences, profound insight, and a sense of ecstasy. Gamma can be fleeting, yet profound.

Throughout labour and birth, you can experience all of these altered states of consciousness. The process of labour itself is intended to pull you out of everyday thinking reality so you can access deeper states of consciousness.

> Basically, so that you can perform a miracle.

Think about this: Can you have an orgasm while thinking about your day? Worrying about the day while you are intimate with your partner rarely results in a fully satisfying sexual experience. This is because you cannot have an orgasm if you are engaged with your thinking rational brain, and if your stress system is activated. Birth is the same.

Most of the environments in which women labour and deliver in do not support the need for engaging in altered state of consciousness. Rather, protocols and procedures interrupt this flow, making it difficult for the woman in labour to remain in that altered state.

If for any reason she perceives her space and experience to be threatening or unsafe, her brain will remain in high alert and the slower frequencies of alpha and theta will be compromised.

Hence, at this stage, it is simply impossible for a mother in labour to surrender to the flow of the event, trust completely in the process, and allow the intensity of labour to overwhelm her so that she can deliver without intervention.

There is nothing wrong with intervention per se. It is not a moral judgment to choose medical assistance. It is, however, destructive if your perception of those interventions is now linked to a belief that 'your body failed you' or that 'you were not strong enough' or that 'you couldn't do it'.

Under such circumstances—fear and stress—your body was working to protect you and your baby by slowing down the process and preventing progression so that you could find 'safety'.

Of course, we do not live in the wild, therefore, rarely do women seek out 'safety' in labour. I have heard of some stories in which women locked themselves in the bathroom at the hospital and delivered on the floor. However, this is rare. Most often women surrender to the lack of control and perceived threats (whether overt or perceived) and note this moment as if they 'gave up'.

Again, I want to impress upon you that you didn't 'give up', but rather, most likely you went into a mode of collapse or immobilization in which your system said 'enough' and started to shut down as a result of too much internalized stress.

The key point here is that you give birth in an altered state of consciousness. Most birthing environments do not support this neurophysiological need. If your stress response was activated and you feared the safety and wellbeing of yourself and your baby, you would have been pulled out of that 'labour-land state'. Labour cannot progress instinctively under such circumstances.

Childbirth professionals are not trained to protect your neurophysiological needs for childbirth. Rather, they are trained to protect you and your baby from dying at all costs.

Why didn't my care provider know this?
Why didn't my care provider protect my neurophysiological needs in labour?
Why did my care provider do what they did?
Why didn't my birthing class teach me the neurophysiological needs of a woman in labour?

These are questions that many of my clients have posed throughout the years. The answer is simple: Because the majority of care providers, such as OB/GYNs, midwives, and family doctors, have not been trained in this paradigm. **They were trained to mitigate risk of death at all cost.**

This means that they were trained to bypass the neurophysiological needs of a mother in labour and to intervene in ways that may be interpreted as traumatic, with the intent to save the life of the baby or the mother. This sounds logical, and for many, they are grateful that these healthcare professionals exist. If an emergency presents, they will be safe.

That said, it is important to understand how this viewpoint is potentially contributing to the rise in obstetrical violence and unnecessary interventions that result in 'birth trauma'. Mothers in labour want to know that they are safe and that their baby is safe. This is expected and instinctive. But at what cost?

There is an underlying belief within the medicalization of childbirth which states that birth is inherently dangerous, and that woman need to be 'saved'.

Such a mindset supports the chronic need to intervene in the process of labour and birth, interrupting that hormonal flow and altered state of consciousness.

This wouldn't necessarily be an issue if it didn't result in millions of women struggling in the postpartum because their nervous systems are now trapped in a trauma response. When the neurophysiological needs of a labouring woman are bypassed because there is a perceived risk of death, the whole environment spins into a state of emergency, triggering adrenaline and cortisol to be released. We know that adrenaline and cortisol (the stress hormones) halt the flow of labouring hormones and can remain trapped in the nervous system as trauma.

If you are reading this book, most likely at some point throughout your experience of labour and birth you were told that 'something is wrong', that an intervention was necessary, and that you or your baby were not doing well. At this point, your needs to feel safe and in control of your environment and body may have been bypassed (at times against your will). In such a case, this moment of 'chaos' and 'emergency' triggers your trauma response, and now you feel like you are watching it all happen from a distance.

Even in emergency situations, the nervous system could be supported immediately after the threat was resolved. This would assist in releasing any stuck energy that is stored and activated within your body. As such, you could complete the trauma response prior to being sent home with your newborn. This could be as simple as helping a mother cry, shake, rage to discharge the stress energy, all the while normalizing that response.

However, because those who are trained as health care professionals are not taught how to support this kind of physiological resolution, women are sent home (or left alone) without the necessary supports in place. This in and of itself can result in the beginning of the challenges in the postpartum that so many mothers face, and that later get labeled as 'postpartum mood disorders'.

The key point here is that most childbirth professionals do not support the neurophysiological needs of a labouring woman. Risk of death trumps the risk of trauma. Postpartum mothers are left to resolve the trauma that is stuck in their nervous system, alone. Very, very few practitioners assess for trauma immediately following birth. Moreover, health care providers are not held accountable for protocols and procedures that can be perceived as violent and invasive.

Birth is an extension of our sexual health and our sexual life.
Trigger warning: This section can trigger past memories and I encourage you to listen to your body and heart and proceed slowly.

When I tell my clients that birth is an extension of their sexual health and their sexuality, they often look at me with bulging eyes. Instinctively, they get it. However, they had not linked it. My guess is that this is because the medicalization of childbirth has done a very good job of separating the two. If in fact we considered this notion, many of the protocols and interventions would be perceived as terribly violating.

And so, creating this separation within our minds has allowed women to tolerate behaviours, under the guise of protocol, that would normally be deemed as abusive, violent, aggressive, and to the extreme, rape.

If we consider the statistic that 1 out of every 3 women has experienced sexual assault of some kind (and there is argument that this is not an accurate representation), we can consider that many women in labour have a history of sexual assault of some kind.

This is a critical point to consider because it is not fully recognized as a potential risk factor in triggering a trauma response in labour. If we consider that, generally speaking, it is more likely that the statistic is closer to 1 out of every 2 women have experienced some form of sexual violation, then every 2nd woman in labour is at risk of having historical information linked to 'feeling unsafe in a vulnerable situation'. This can flare up throughout labour and birth.

If we consider the mere fact that women in general have been oppressed for eons and, under the global dominant worldview, are still secondary to men, it is plausible that just being in a vulnerable position will trigger a sense of 'being out of control' or a 'handing over of power'. This sounds like: *They are right, I am wrong.*

If we consider that women of colour, Indigenous women, marginalized women, Muslim women and low-income women are further oppressed under the governing system at large, then they are at even greater risk of being violated, losing power, and being the victims of overt violence in labour.

As you can see, separating childbirth from our sexual health or sexuality has allowed women to continue to be placed in vulnerable positions where an 'other' has power over them.

If you're having the type of *a-ha* moment that I did when I connected these ideas, than you also may be feeling anger or even rage. I know I sure felt enraged when I recognized that women are being violated during childbirth under the guise of 'safety'.

If you can relate to this conversation, please know that you can heal. It was not 'all your fault'. The system is broken (we know this) and the mainstream childbirth environment rarely supports the sanctity of childbirth as an extension of your sexual health. It also doesn't consider your body as a sacred temple that has carried and created life. This lack of respect and consideration has given permission to care givers, of all genders, to violate without consent and have power over women in labour.

The key point here is: under such circumstances is it any wonder that women's bodies are 'failing to progress' in labour? That women cannot push their babies out under distress? That women feel humiliated and silenced? That women are at risk of experiencing trauma during birth? That women feel further disconnected from their bodies and sexuality after giving birth? And that, when they are told that there was something wrong with their body or their baby, they believe it was all their fault?

I invite you to begin to explore these deeper questions about your childbirth experience. Most mothers remember accurately what was happening throughout their pregnancy, labour and delivery. Please take the time to reflect and feel into your previous birth experience and pay attention to the smaller details of when you first started to question your ability to give birth the way you had hoped.

REFLECTIVE EXERCISE
ON ANGER AND BLAME

When did the 'chaos' start happening?

At what point did you stop feeling safe in labour? Did you ever 'feel' safe?

When did you first start to experience doubt in your labour?

What or who were you doubting?

What did your doubt voice sound like?

What happened after you started to doubt?

What shifted for you when your doubt surfaced?

What do you wish you had known or done differently once the doubt set in?

What did your labouring-self need that was not provided?
How did you need to be supported at that time?

THERAPEUTIC ACTIVITY
Narrative Exercise

This activity encourages you to explore your feelings associated with doubt and disappointment. You just learned a lot about the need for safety and trust in labour, and you explored questions pertaining to doubt throughout your experience of labour and birth. In this exercise, I invite you to consider the following question.

When I think about my childbirth experience now, I am still feeling [...] because...

CHAPTER 9

LEARNING TO SEE THINGS DIFFERENTLY

"A thought is harmless unless we believe it. It's not our thoughts, but our attachment to our thoughts, that causes suffering. Attaching to a thought means believing that it's true, without inquiring. A belief is a thought that we've been attaching to, often for years." ~ Byron Katie

The Power of Perception

Consider the following:
- ★ Perception is powerful.
- ★ You tell yourself something about every situation.
- ★ You tell yourself something about YOURSELF as it pertains to a situation.
- ★ Your mind can be both a wonderful and a destructive tool.
- ★ Perceiving your childbirth through a different lens is within your control.
- ★ The brain is a meaning-making organ.
- ★ The brain seeks to make sense out of the senseless.
- ★ How you tell your story indicates how much you have healed.
- ★ Awareness is key.
- ★ Without insight, it is difficult to heal.
- ★ Humans search for meaning in the chaos and the pain.
- ★ You are more than your thoughts and beliefs, and more than your pain.
- ★ You can become aware of your thoughts, question them, and choose to not believe them.
- ★ Stressful thoughts give rise to painful feelings, give rise to state of being.
- ★ We perceive through the lens of our past until we become conscious of it.

Over the years I have attended numerous pieces of training on trauma recovery, along with an incessant drive to consume information about the topic. I was driven to understand my diagnosis of PTSD and to unearth how I can heal. This drive led me to finish grad school, train as a trauma-informed therapist and develop this healing program for mothers.

I think what inspires me the most about becoming trauma-informed is the power gained. I knew in my bones that I could heal. And I hold this belief for others as well. In my past, I struggled with depression for years, and I felt disempowered and afraid of being diagnosed with a mental illness. I held a perception that it meant that I would be cursed forever.

I tried to change my thoughts, so I could feel better. However, I didn't experience the results I craved. Granted, this quest to 'change my thinking' helped me become mindfully attuned to my thoughts. And as it stands, mindfulness is now receiving gold star status in healing and recovery.

Our physiology is innately intelligent and has a drive that 'seeks' to attune towards health. I love this about our bodies. Our mind is deeply interconnected to our physiology (for those eager to unpack the concept of the mind, read *The Mind* by Dan Siegel).

The body and mind are one
and it is about time that we claim this knowing.

It makes sense that both the physiological *and* psychological impacts of the event ought to be a part of the trauma discourse. The literature readily available today surmounts what was available just six years ago. It is as if trauma-informed care has skyrocketed. I imagine it has done so because it speaks to how we can heal tangibly. It offers a perspective on causation to many of today's mental, emotional, physical, relational and behavioural challenges—not just a list of symptoms but a probable physiological cause due to unprocessed traumatic material in the nervous system.

Within the conversation of trauma-informed care, we recognize that each person is impacted by a traumatic event differently and each person has different variables to consider. **One of the variables concerns how the experience becomes etched into the mind/memory/psyche of the individual. In other words,** *how the individual perceives the event.*

This comment has left me with many questions. A somewhat simple statement is full of complicated calculations and considerations:

What is perception?
How is perception formed?

How do we control perception? Or do we?
How do we change perception?
Who is in control—the self or the brain?
Who is the self?

As you can imagine, this spiraled me down a rabbit hole of deeper discovery, philosophical consideration, spiritual questioning and scientific evidence. Unpacking the notion of perception is not an easy task. There is little room for error because misrepresenting a concept could send the reader down the wrong rabbit hole.

And yet, isn't it all perception anyway? By that I mean the lens through which you read this has perceptions embedded within it—'filters'. This leaves one to pose the following question: *What are those filters made of?*

Definition of Perception
Perception, according to the Apple dictionary refers to

> *1. the ability to see, hear, or become aware of something through the senses. The neurophysiological processes, including memory, by which an organism becomes aware of and interprets external stimuli.*
> *2. the way in which something is regarded, understood, or interpreted. An intuitive understanding and insight.*

Thus, perception is the process in which we make sense out of an event. It includes our thoughts and senses. Perception informs how we communicate about an experience, both externally and internally. We are meaning-making machines.

For some time now, I would argue that we were taught that we have free will and, thus, how we understand and interpret an experience is within our realm of control. And so, if it is within our power to influence how we perceive an experience, then do we have control over how we make sense out of an event? Regardless if the event is positive or traumatic.

This above notion may sound optimistic and perhaps even motivating for some. And when I first considered this idea, I felt empowered to do something about my state of being. That said, the deeper I went down the rabbit hole, the more challenged I became by this concept.

First of all, I felt frustrated that I encoded my traumatic events in a negative way that complicated my healing and my physiological response to trauma. I experienced self-blame. Why is it that some people could move on and have a less aggravating perception of an event, while others become entirely derailed by the experience? Could perception be the main differentiating factor?

Let me offer an example specific to the demographic I most often serve:

Mother 1—Came to therapy because she had an unplanned, unwanted C-section after a transfer to hospital for complications that could have been terminal for either herself or her newborn. She was relatively calm about the event. She was processing some grief due to the loss of her physical constitution and her dream birth, but otherwise had a healthy perspective that a C-section was the best option at the time. It made sense to her. She felt sad about the event, but grateful to be a mother. She expressed frustration that she didn't plan for a C-section or complications, and felt annoyed with herself, but said: "It was needed. I am well. My baby is well. We will be okay". After a few sessions of grief therapy, the mother felt like she had made sense of the experience and in her words: "I am okay with what happened." She wasn't showing signs of dysregulated physiology, and one would assess that she was not carrying any trauma about this event, even though her life and her baby's life had been threatened.

Her perception was that: "I am okay. My baby is okay. It is over now. We are okay. It makes sense to me. It is okay to have disappointment and grief, and I will move on."

Mother 2—Came to therapy because of an unplanned, unwanted C-section after a transfer to the hospital for 'failure to progress' and a drop in the baby's heart rate. Everything about the event felt horrifying to her. The image I got was that of a battleground. She felt the terror that her baby was unsafe. She didn't want to be cut open. She didn't trust the hospital staff, and she didn't trust the midwives. She presented as dysregulated, hyperaroused, disorientated, and had big energy and emotions. It seems as though she was about to explode or float out of the room. She had difficulty maintaining eye contact and wanted to tell me her story over and over again. One of the themes she brought up several times was that the caregivers failed her. She perceived the event as disempowering, disrespectful, disheartening, and she believed that the caregivers were to blame.

Her perception was that: "I was harmed. I was violated. I was mistreated. It is all their fault. I was neglected."

Although these are radically different examples, they are based on similar starting points. Both mothers experienced unwanted C-sections, transfers to the hospital, and a threat to their baby's wellbeing. Both suffered physical trauma due to surgery (according to Levine, surgery is a trauma) and each would have experienced prolonged pain due to an induction at some point throughout their labour.

Both mothers were equally at risk of having experienced their birth as traumatic based on these factors. However, both had different experiences and processed differently in the postpartum. Recovery has been quicker for Mother 1. Mother 2 presented with symptoms of postpartum PTSD. All of which poses the question: *Why did Mother 2 imprint her birth as traumatic? Did she have control over this? Does she have the power to change her perception of the event?* These are hard questions to consider.

By no means does it reflect that Mother 1 is 'behaving' better than Mother 2. A trap that the old worldview can feed is one that says: *Just get over it and get on with it. It is selfish to focus on the self.* This old worldview leaves mothers feeling ashamed and guilty for how they are responding to their childbirth and can result in suppression of emotions and thoughts. This simply does not work because your physiology won't forget about it. As Van Der Kolk states: "Your body keeps the score". Unfortunately, there is no ignoring emotions; there is only going through them.

There are so many variables that could have contributed to each of the mothers' experiences of birth. Some factors to consider include:
- ★ History of attachment with family of origin.
- ★ Adverse childhood experiences (abuse, neglect, poverty, malnutrition).
- ★ History of oppression (marginalized race, gender, religion).
- ★ Financial stress.
- ★ History of sexual assault.
- ★ Nutrition.
- ★ Support systems.
- ★ Religious or spiritual beliefs.
- ★ Physical health before birth.
- ★ Mental health before birth.
- ★ Marital status and relationship health.
- ★ Other stressors.

All of these reasons (and more) influence a person's 'way of being' in the world. Further, they inform how our physiology and psychology encodes (make sense of) life events. Unless we become conscious of this material intrinsically, we cannot 'change' our way of thinking and being. However, can we control how we perceive an event *at the time of the event?* Or is it only afterwards that we can influence how we store the information?

From what I believe, our past informs our present way of being until we wake up to our programs of the past. If we are unconscious of how our past experiences have influenced our way of thinking, feeling, doing, and being, then we have no power to change our perception of an event.

Perception is how we make sense of a life event. **And how we make sense of current circumstances is based on our past experiences.** Therefore, we are living in the past until we become conscious of these core patterned ways of being. Dr. Joe Dispenza speaks powerfully about this notion in his book *Breaking the Habit of Being Yourself*.

We cannot escape life without experiencing traumatic events or adversities. Granted, some are more horrific than others. However, from what we understand, humans have been suffering from trauma as far back as we go. We have a physiological system that responds to trauma and fights for our survival. The problem is that once we have 'survived', unlike other mammals, humans have a hard time returning to a state of calmness and cohesiveness. The challenge is that our neocortex—the thinking brain—gets in the way.

We have a thinking brain that tries to make sense out of every act and experience. This brain is responsible for our evolution and, also, **it keeps us trapped in trauma as we relive it in our mind's eye over and over again.** It is as if trauma glitches the system for some and puts the record on repeat. Thankfully, there are ways in which we can recover and respond to glitches in the system.

It is imperative that the trauma response completes its instinctive cycle. Thus, body-centered therapies are beneficial. They can move the trapped energy in the nervous system. Associated with this nervous system energy are all the thoughts, emotions, felt sensations and images about the event. Those also need to be processed, and 'digested' so that the limbic system can turn off the alarm bells.

During this process, I am noticing that the final phase of recovery pertains to a change in perception in which the person views the situation from a different vantage point. Usually this involves a compassionate release towards self and other.

This does not mean that if someone experienced violence and violation that the perpetrator should not be held accountable for their harmful actions or that a mother should not file a complaint against a caregiver if deemed necessary. But instead, the perceptual field grows to include deeper understanding of the self at that time, the others at that time, and any influencing historical information that would elicit a compassionate tone of understanding.

Does this sound like a spiritual awakening?

From my perspective that is exactly what is happening when we grow from one state of perception to another that includes the self, the other, all living creatures, our planet, and the cosmos. In a state of deep understanding, we bypass our conditioned responses based on historical content. Our physiology may 'keep the score', but one can argue that 'consciousness' exists within and without the physiology.

When we can 'know' that we are more than our physiology and more than the programs we have received through genetics and experiences, then we can begin to change our embedded reactionary responses to life events—be they traumatic or ecstatic.

For many, trauma is a wake-up call to move beyond our physiology. We cannot do anything about our past experiences, *but we can change how we think and feel about them.* When faced with a traumatic event, we may not be able to influence how our system responds to that experience; our physiology responds quicker than our thinking brain can. It is as if we are always one step behind the body's imprinted and instinctive reactions. So, how can we catch up?

This leads me to pose a question about consciousness itself or, rather, the part of the self that is the Witness, the spiritual self, the higher self, the One, the Void. Perhaps The Buddha was on to something as a contemplative enlightened figure who speaks about the cycle of human suffering. He speaks about transcending suffering by non-attachment to the ego identity. I hear: un-attachment to our physiology.

Our physiology holds our imprinted ways of thinking, feeling and doing. When traced back all the way to the wombs of our mothers, we know that chemicals tell us if we are safe, wanted, secure, loved. These chemicals are already being embedded into our growing embryo.

We learn about the external world before we are born via our mother's response to it. One could argue that we are born imprinted with pertinent information about our place in the world. From there we learn about our physical self through relational attunement with our primary caregivers.

Before we can make sense rationally, we are receiving perceptions about belonging, safety, love, pain, emotions and behaviour. We mirror those around us. Our personality emerges from these experiences. I liken my personality to a large dose of environmental circumstances infused with the energetics of my 'soul'. Much of how I perceive myself is based on external circumstances that informed me about myself, before the age of seven. From here we see the birth of 'core beliefs' and, in particular, core limiting beliefs.

> Our perceptions are infused with core beliefs
> about the self, others, and ways of being in the world.

Thus, going back to the earlier example about the two different mothers, one could postulate that Mother 1 holds a core belief based on historical experiences: *"I am okay in the world, it is safe to be here."* Whereas, it is possible that Mother 2 holds a core belief based on historical experiences: *"The world is unsafe, and I am at risk of being harmed."*

I am painting with broad strokes with this last statement. However, I am offering a point of view that how we currently perceive aspects of our history can profoundly influence a traumatic experience in ways we have not considered before.

Secondly, **I am suggesting that trauma is an opportunity for awakening to the 'self' that exists outside of our physiology**. As such, perhaps from this place, we can rewire how we store memories so that we are no longer chasing our physiological reactions, but instead 'changing the program' so that the physiology responds differently in the future. Is this not what the ancients meant when they said: *When you heal, you heal seven generations back and seven generations forward?*

Two powerful questions to help you access your core beliefs are:

> What am I telling myself about the situation—
> what am I hearing myself say to myself about the situation?

> What am I telling myself about *myself* as it pertains to the situation—
> what does this mean about *me* as a person?

Trauma and The Perception of Pain in Labour

What follows is an email exchange I had recently with a mother. The email exchange is included with her consent because I think it illustrates important points.

Based on the limited information I had about this mother initially, I understood that she was pregnant with her fourth child and generally had a history of satisfied births and deliveries. However, during her third pregnancy she experienced emotional trauma related to something else, which impacted her early labour experience and resulted in increased pain with contractions.

She reached out because she was noticing she was reliving this emotional trauma and she was afraid of the onset of labour.

Her questions were:
1. I'm looking for information on the connection between experiencing OTHER trauma and going into labour / giving birth and the affect it can have on your pain perception / pain threshold DURING labour.
2. I found out that going through trauma can in fact lower your pain threshold (with other pain, not the pain from the trauma) and cause the pain you experience to be more intense. Is there any information on this that will help to prepare myself and to help myself be less scared of what is to come?
3. I also feel like I'm going through the same trauma again—just not as intense as when it happened. Is there anything I can do to work through this?

Let's examine this closer.

The first theme that arises is her history of previous trauma (unrelated to birth) and the potential impact on labour and delivery. Trauma is pervasive, period. The symptoms of a traumatic stress response can yield its ugly head at any point, especially if we are engaged in stressful or vulnerable events. That said, I want to highlight the resilience and grit factor that humans demonstrate over and over again. The bottom line is that we can tolerate an enormous amount of adversity and continue to thrive. Truly, this is amazing.

We all have a tipping point. As humans we can tolerate a lot, however, **all of a sudden one adverse experience can tip the scale** and we present with symptoms of the traumatic stress response. As previously mentioned, unresolved historical trauma can increase your risk of childbirth trauma. However, there are so many variable factors to consider. **Each mother has vulnerabilities and strengths, and in any given moment, anything can change. Our *perception* of the event is as powerful as the event itself.**

This is why two people can experience the same traumatic event and one may develop post-traumatic stress symptoms while the other returns to a state of health after a debrief and a good cry/shake/laugh/roar.

What does 'resolving' trauma mean?
Simply put, has your emotional debris been felt and integrated? Has it been grieved? Has your brain stored the event properly so that it is no longer flooding your system with unprocessed emotional material? Has your nervous system been restored to homeostasis, in such that it no longer perceives your current reality as threatening? Has your body released the trauma through movement, sound, expression and felt sensations? Have you made sense out of the situation?

Have you applied meaning to the event? Do you feel safe in your body and in your environment?

These are all questions to consider when trying to resolve or heal from trauma. We do know that healing from one adverse event is less complicated than healing from a history of multiple traumatic events. That said, the process is similar regardless and contemplating these questions, and receiving necessary support to facilitate movement through the process, is helpful.

What can happen during labour and delivery?

As we learned earlier, labour and delivery is a physiologically and emotionally stressful event for any mother. During this experience mothers are vulnerable albeit powerful. **This vulnerability can result in the triggering of a 'trauma' response (a toxic stress response) in that the mother does not feel safe, perceives the situation as harmful to baby or herself, does not trust the caregivers and perceives an utter lack of control.**

If the historical traumatic event or episodes have not been processed, integrated, and healed, it is possible that the mother's system can become activated, as above, and become flooded with adrenaline ('gas') and cortisol ('brakes'). Both of these are counterproductive to the progression of labour. These hormones can halt or prolong the labouring experience, which lends to the second theme on perceived pain.

Turning back to the email exchange: the second theme we see arise is around the mother's perception of pain and ability to tolerate labour pain. Frederick Leboyer, a grandfather obstetrician who wrote *Birth Without Violence,* spoke about the pain-perception cycle being connected to an increase in perceived fear.

The cycle is as such:

$$\text{Fear} = \text{Tension} = \text{Pain}$$
$$\text{Pain} = \text{Fear} = \text{Tension}$$

As such, if a mother perceives her environment as unsafe or out of control for any reason, or if she feels something in her body that links to a memory of past violation or pain, her autonomic nervous system will move into high gear and flood her system with adrenaline (the hormone associated with fight or flight).

Cortisol is a secondary hormone that comes online in attempt to counterbalance the rush of adrenaline. With both cortisol and adrenaline flooding the system, the body constricts and retracts in an attempt to protect itself from perceived harm. This constriction results in tension. And, tension increases pain.

When we are constricting, in attempt to avoid pain, we are resisting the natural pain of labour, thus intensifying the experience of labour pain. The antidote is counterintuitive: to move towards the pain, not away from it. And to challenge the intrusive fearful thoughts. In other words, is the fear rational or perceived? The battle with labour is often the dance between moving towards pain yet wanting to run away and resist it.

So, what is a mother to do? Sometimes knowing too much complicates matters. Fearing the 'potential' triggers during labour and birth because we know that unresolved trauma may contribute to more painful or complicated labour, only adds fuel to the fire.

I remember one of my teachers, Dr. Michel Odent, saying that mothers need to get out of their thinking brain. And caregivers need to do whatever it takes to reduce potential stressors.

There is much that a mother can do in preparation:
- ★ Receive trauma-informed counselling to process emotions
- ★ Speak to your caregivers openly about your fears and history
- ★ Question, challenge and flow your fears
- ★ Ensure that you trust your caregivers
- ★ Seek out practitioners who believe in informed consent
- ★ Educate yourself about the holistic stages of labour and birth as an altered-state experience (www.thematrona.com)
- ★ Engage in transparent communication between your caregiver, family and friends
- ★ Move your body through yoga, dance, walk and play
- ★ Learn how to support your nervous system when it is activated
- ★ Engage in creative activities
- ★ Write in a journal
- ★ Develop a spiritual or meditative practice
- ★ Do what you can to build trust in your body and the process of birth
- ★ Foster loving supportive relationships

Is there a silver lining? Yes. Human beings and mothers are resilient. We can heal, and we can heal during labour and birth.

If the pain is unbearable, do what is most compassionate in that moment. Sometimes the most compassionate choice is pain medication. Love and self-compassion are powerful medicines and are antidotes to trauma. Human beings are wired for love (if you're interested in this topic, I encourage you to read writing by Stan Tatkin or Stephen Porges).

> Giving birth is an act of selfless courageous love,
> regardless of how we deliver our babies.

REFLECTIVE EXERCISE
BUILDING COMPASSION

"What if, first, we got clear on how we actually wanted to feel in our life, and then we laid out our intentions? What if your most desired feelings consciously informed how you plan your day, your year, your career, your holidays—your life?" ~Danielle LaPorte

You have come this far and braved some deep waters. You have experienced your grief, your anger, your doubt and shame. You have named it and inquired deep within. You have demonstrated a profound desire to engage in your healing process.

You may be tired, distressed or even ready to quit the process. **Perhaps it feels like you are at the precipice of change; the transitional stage of healing.** Or maybe, you don't see the point of feeling into all these uncomfortable feelings.

Now is the time to hold onto something so powerful within, a deep trust in this process that is unfolding, so you can continue to engage with a full heart ablaze.

To begin, take a moment and remind yourself 'why' you chose to heal.
Drop into your heart and feel into your desire. Take note and set an intention before moving forward. Hold yourself and this process with utmost care and kindness. Explore how you *want* to feel about your birth experience.

Ask the question:
How do you *want* to feel about your childbirth experience?

When it comes to my childbirth experience, I want to feel...

When it comes to myself as a mother, I want to feel...

Now, can you imagine what it would be like if you embraced those feelings?

REFLECTIVE EXERCISE
REVISITING YOUR WHY

"When we hang onto our past, we cannot move into our future in a newfound way. Our past determines our present and our future." ~ Dr. Joe Dispenza

The following exercise invites you to reflect upon your Why again. Go back to the beginning of this guidebook (page xvii) and re-read your notes from the first reflective exercise.

Why are you choosing to engage in your healing and move into the discomforts of the healing emotions? Why are you working so hard?

What is (or has been) your anchor—the belief or motivation that is keeping you above water?

The pain of labour is obvious. You receive your newborn on the other side of the intense journey. The pain of healing is not so obvious. What do you hope to receive on the other side of this journey?

What are you afraid to let go of?
What part of your birth story do you want to hold onto?

CHAPTER 10

Exploring Meaning in Motherhood

"The most important 'job' on this planet is raising our next generation with loving, attuned, presence and meaningful connection." ~ Jennifer Summerfeldt

On Integration and The Postpartum

In psychology, integration is a key component of mental health and overall health. When we make sense of our life circumstances, feel our emotions that have been trapped in our body, and flow a coherent story about our life without a huge amount of activation, it is said that we have integrated an experience.

Thus, we can weave this story into the tapestry of our life, giving rise to our individual humanity. Some stories carry more weight, requiring more time to integrate. Yet, usually those experiences are turning points throughout our life that mold and shape our character.

Childbirth is one of these kinds of experiences—rich in meaning and gravitas. Hence, when a woman gives birth, regardless of her birth experience and outcome, she holds a very precious story that will forever be etched into her psyche and cells. This process of unfolding, uncovering, undoing, reclaiming, remembering and reorienting, is and never was intended to be rushed.

We rush the postpartum.

When a mother is rushed in her postpartum or holds an impression that she should somehow get it 'together' and 'get back to a normal way of being and doing', she is most likely going to be faced with struggles in her postpartum. Those struggles can show up as depression and anxiety.

Is it possible that a mother's intelligent system is screaming at her to pay attention, to slow down and listen, and that something is off balance? Why are we so quick to label our experience as 'something' and get this label from someone who is an 'expert' in the field? Rather, what if we were encouraged to drop in and listen to what the symptoms are saying? And, be supported to follow through on this listening?

Allow me to elaborate. Having experienced my own three postpartums, and witnessed many others, there are a few things that I have noticed. After a woman has given birth she is in an altered state of consciousness, which causes her to get a felt sense of being between 'worlds' or 'realities'. It is not always obvious and because our everyday experience rarely courts the altered state of consciousness, it can feel very foreign and unfamiliar to some moms. Even if the mother does not 'feel' this in-between state, something in her *knows* that *something* is or should be different.

A miracle took place, albeit an everyday miracle, but a miracle of creation. And why is it that we are so quick to close this state of awe? Granted all the attention goes towards the baby and receiving the baby, and sometimes the mother is left to her own accord and neglected. Society grants very little attention and reverence to what the mother just experienced—let alone the fact that she sacrificed her body, in an act of love, for the past nine months.

> She just delivered a baby (a human),
> from a water to an earth environment,
> *and she is expected to have it all figured out within a few weeks?*

There are so many physical changes that are taking place in the immediate postpartum that use up a lot of vital energy. For example: The mother's uterus changes shape and size and shifts from being the size of a watermelon to that of a pear again; her hormones change and are needed to produce milk; her blood volume goes back to normal after doubling in quantity; her organs go back into 'place' within the body; if she had surgery, she is healing an incision; if she had damage to her pelvic floor, she is healing her tissue; if she lost blood, she is rebuilding blood volume; she is regaining vitality after giving all her nutrients to the growing fetus for the past nine months; she is replenishing her energy after exerting it during labour and delivery; she is resting after staying up for hours upon hours during a long labour.

As you can imagine there are many physiological adjustments and changes taking place that would exhaust anyone. And standard care suggests that it takes six weeks to return to 'pre-pregnancy' mode. First of all, there is no such thing as pre-pregnancy or going back to that. Secondly, none of these physiological changes address the psychological, emotional, relational and spiritual/energetic changes that occurred. **Mothers also need time for integration.**

Childbirth is a woman's vision quest.

Much about modern obstetrics and midwifery lacks regard to this notion. And, the largest implication is the lack of regard to the sacred act of giving birth— the dismembering of birth and the compartmentalizing of that which cannot be compartmentalized.

As a keeper of birth stories, I have heard and read hundreds. These stories have included everything from orgasmic birthing experiences to violent, traumatic events. In all of these stories there is a common thread: **All of these women *knew* that they were experiencing something profound, life altering and other-worldly.**

Foundationally, every woman who has shared her story has been deeply imprinted by that event. It is etched into her cells and her psyche. **Our lack of reverence, culturally, for the experience of birth is in my opinion showing up in the postpartum.**

Somehow, many mothers get the impression like they are supposed to just sort it all out in a short period of time. Get over the event. And have it all figured out— nursing, night sleeping, crying, diapering, illness, development—as if they are born into being a professional mother. Each baby requires time and attention to nurture the unique relational bond between each family member. There is no right way or one way, but there is a unique way.

On top of the pressure to have it all figured out within a certain time frame, there is the added pressure to take on a new 'job' as an at-home mother which includes cleaning, cooking, organizing, socializing and tending to the baby. I have heard over and over again mothers express guilt connected to the concept that they 'should' be doing more around the house now that they are home or that they are failures because they can't 'keep it in order'.

Can you sense the tension building in any mother's experience of the postpartum?

If for some reason a mother is challenged to have all of this figured out within the first few weeks or months after giving birth, and if her body is not healing as 'normal', and if she is struggling with sleep, colic, illness or nursing, one can understand how her nervous system would be absolutely taxed. Thus contributing to the onset of postpartum mood challenges—anxiety and/or depressive states. But there is more, not only has her nervous system gone array, she is dying on a soul level.

Let us add one more challenge that many mothers face in the postpartum: **isolation and loneliness.**

As previously discussed, motherhood can be a very isolating experience. Part of this is because many mothers are exhausted and adding a social engagement to the mix is just too much. Sometimes, mothers have expressed feeling too ashamed to connect with other mothers because they are struggling. This isolation is a result of our nuclear family structure which has separated us from community and connection. Motherhood was never intended to be a role that is 'performed' in an isolated environment.

All of these factors impact the postpartum mother's process of integration. Further, when a mother's primary partner and closest family members feed a mythical tale—that she is supposed to be better by now, have it all figured out, hide or tone down her emotions, take on many jobs and do them well, be happy, love her children, have a nice clean home, nourish her family, work towards getting her pre-pregnancy body back—she is likely to go *'mad'*.

> Both 'mad' in the sense of a psychic wild pain
> and 'mad' in the sense of rage.

I would argue that this rage is necessary and insightful. It is a collective rage that is screaming *'something is terribly wrong about what is happening'*. This rage is shared, and I can attest to this because I have both experienced it and witnessed it in hundreds of women. Most often however, this rage is never given space to be witnessed. There is fear that this rage will either:
   a. harm another or the self; or
   b. cause one to be sent to a mental institution.

Sadly, when we explore the depths of this fear, usually these are the two fears that prevent a mother from moving into this sacred rage.

Women are not allowed to rage. Period.

We are led to believe that it is dangerous. Too much. Violent. Aggressive. Wrong. Bad. Mean. Denotes a lack of control.

What happens when mothers are not encouraged to voice and do something with their rage? It turns into anxiety or depression or, in some horrific cases, psychosis.

What would being held in a manner that fosters integration offer mothers?

- ★ Space to *speak* about the fullness of their perinatal experience.
- ★ Space to emote and *feel* into the fullness of this experience.
- ★ Time to collect her *pieces* that have just been totally discombobulated throughout pregnancy and birth.
- ★ Time to reorient and *reconnect* to herself, her baby, her loved ones.
- ★ Nourishment both physically and soulfully.
- ★ Space to create *meaning* from this life changing experience.
- ★ A *knowing* that she does not have to have it all together or figured out, and that there is no pressure for her to be a certain way or do certain things.
- ★ A *trust* in the process and in herself as a mother.

Healing.

REFLECTIVE EXERCISE
ON THE POSTPARTUM

I invite you to contemplate these questions. Share them with others or keep them close to your heart. **Begin conversations with other mothers in your community about any or all of these concepts presented.** Change will only happen when mothers claim something different for themselves. When collectively we begin to speak about the 'unspeakable' aspects of the childbirth continuum. When the sacred is included in the conversations about birth and postpartum. And when the rage is acknowledged and understood.

How did you rush your postpartum 'recovery'?

How did the people around you rush your postpartum?

What were you in a rush to do? What were you rushing? Why were you rushing?

Are you rushing to get back to normal? What normal? What was your concept of normal? Who defined 'normal' anyways? Is there anything 'normal' about the way we live?

What were the consequences of rushing your postpartum?

What expectations were placed upon you, both internally and externally?

What do you still need to begin to integrate the fullness of your childbirth experience?

What is/was being asked of you?

What would you like to say to those you love, to other mothers, or to the world that you know would shift something for you and other mothers?

What was lacking in your postpartum? What was off?

What is your rage or grief about?

On Mindfulness and Motherhood

Mindfulness is a practice of noticing and observing that which is arising within one's internal space, in any given moment, without judgment or analysis. **Although, I love the simplicity of this act of kindness towards oneself, I must acknowledge the difficulty involved in training the mind to become mindful as a mother.**

If you are anything like me, you might agree with my long-held frustration towards the mindfulness movement being dominated by mostly a masculine point of view.

Don't get me wrong: I appreciate all the teachings and the plethora of research about the benefits of having a practice of mindfulness. And, I acknowledge the wisdom that these wise men have offered us—His Holiness the Dalai Lama, Ram Dass, Dan Siegel, Ron Siegel, Jon Kabat-Zinn, Deepak Chopra, Thich Nhat Hanh, Joe Dispenza and Ken Wilber—to name a few. **That said, as a mother, woman, and feminist, I have struggled over the years to embody the teachings of these masters because, well, they just don't fit in with modern motherhood.**

Since I was 13 years-old I have attempted to integrate a practice of meditation into my daily life for stress reduction as an athlete, to deal with symptoms of depression, and to find solace as a mother. The literature and current research clearly state the benefits of a daily practice of mindfulness. In an attempt to alleviate my daily struggles with depression, motherhood and marriage, I figured a practice of meditation would offer much sought-after relief.

Needless to say, I struggled to include this isolated practice into my life as a mother, and I often felt like a failure. I tried waking up earlier, staying up later, listening to guided meditations, using binaural beats, engaging in shamanic journeying, and even participating with shamanic medicines.

Today, my children are teenagers and I have more space for uninterrupted time to include a practice, yet I still find myself jealous of my friends without kids who can sit in meditation for 1-2 hours a day or go away on week-long retreats.

Can you sense the groaning frustration?

I held a perception that these practices only benefit those who can find the time and space for them throughout a day. Let's face it, motherhood is all-encompassing and rarely gives rise to the space needed for such a practice. Sure, 20 minutes a day sounds doable. But when mothers struggle to merely take a shower, how are they supposed to find time for a 20-minute sit? Further, new mothers are chronically sleep-deprived and by the time the day comes to a close they are most likely to crash with their kids or zone out in front of Netflix to have a 'break' from the day. I get it, I have been there.

My intention is not to tell mothers that they 'should' give up Netflix and instead choose a practice of mindfulness because that would be better for them. Mothers have enough 'should-ing' in a day. The last thing we need is another 'should' that adds to our already critical mindset that lets us know all the ways in which we are 'not good enough' as mothers.

It is as if the 'not good enough' voice is amplified when we become mothers, and our children let us know on a daily basis all the areas in which we are 'failing'. Although this negative perception of self-as-mother is almost always inaccurate, I have yet to meet a mother who is not challenged by a negative self-perception of motherhood.

Would mindfulness help quiet this internal critical voice? Most likely, yes. But... But for some reason knowing this is not motivating enough to figure out a way to engage in a daily practice of mindfulness. I would argue the reason is twofold:

    a. The Western worldview of modern motherhood does not support this aspect of self-care, and

    b. the recommended practice is not realistic for today's mother.

Let's take a look at these two statements.

Challenge A: the Western worldview of modern motherhood does not support this aspect of self-care.

As a therapist, the field itself often focuses on 'self-care'. *"What do you do for self-care?"* is a common question posed to mothers in the postpartum, holding up an assumption that if mothers took more time for themselves they would be happier and more balanced. **Most mothers can relate to the fact that when their children are babies, taking a shower without interruption is an arduous task.** Let alone staying on top of the 'to-do' list that many mothers create in their heads.

Realistically, a day and life of a new mother consists of changing diapers, feeding, dealing with a crying infant, maybe taking a nap, figuring out food needs, and finally, collapsing in bed to be awoken within a few hours to do the whole thing over again throughout the night (and add subsequent children to the mix, and well, it is a gong show). I recall Dr. Sears stating in his 'Dr. Sears Baby Book' something to the tune that a mother's clock is a 24-hour clock and the routine that you were once accustomed to is no longer available. Motherhood is a 24/7 job. **As our children grow, the demands may change but the pull to be 'on' 24/7 doesn't.**

To top it all off, the role of motherhood is viewed as an aside; an adjunct to the role of a contributing citizen (i.e., working in the job force). This mindset festers in the minds of many mothers with thoughts like: "I am not contributing enough," "I am a failure because I am not earning a living," or "I need to manage it all—career and motherhood." Finding meaning in motherhood is an arduous task for many. What is certain is that most mothers would agree that they love their children.

And to complicate matters, mothers who face discrimination and/or abuse, oppression due to race or religion, or find themselves marginalized in any manner, experience a multitude of challenges. **These added stressors, atop an already stressful situation (motherhood), pose additional challenges that would cause any mother to scoff at the notion that 'mindfulness' would be beneficial.** Survival is the key motivator in such circumstances. Thus, acknowledging that the mere fact that a mother can contemplate how to include a practice of mindfulness into their daily lives, is a privileged conversation.

Considering these general challenges faced by modern mothers, is it any wonder why self-care takes a back burner? Women have been informed for a long while now, based upon perceptions of roles in society, that 'others' come before their needs.

The perception of 'The Good Mother' is one of a nurturing, loving, care provider, who tends to the home and hearth. And often within this archetypal framework, the mother is also the martyr or the giver of all that she has (including her life in childbirth for some) until her inner well is empty.

HOW CAN WE BALANCE THIS DEEPLY INGRAINED CONCEPT OF 'THE GOOD MOTHER' WITH REALITY?

Further, how can we include self-care behaviours and boundaries pertaining to time, individuality, health, passion, and identity? Introducing the practice of mindfulness requires a kind of reorganizing. It is not as simple as stating: "You need merely to include a 20-minute practice daily, with discipline, in order for you to feel better'. Statements like this ignite the critical voice that keeps us feeling small and ashamed.

Compounding the challenge is that many of the men who speak about mindfulness do so from a place that is informed by their experiences of life as a man. Not life as a mother.

Instead, I propose that the notion of self-care and mindfulness should take on a different, mother-inspired approach, one that speaks a new language and no longer fuels the fear of 'not good enough'.

Challenge B: the recommended practice is not realistic for today's mother.

When will I find the time? This is the pressing question. **The answers:** wake up earlier, go to bed later, be selfish with your time, if you want it bad enough you will find the time. The list goes on and on. Often this leaves a mother to believe that if she doesn't do those things then she has failed somehow. In some cases, it causes her to give up completely.

I know this place all too well. I struggled with this throughout my journey as a mother of three children. I knew that the mental health benefits of practicing meditation would lend to a mindful way of being. And yet, I wrestled with finding time for just me. When I finally had some time alone, I wanted to get out of the house and go for coffee with friends, or just fall asleep. I didn't want to spend that time alone, in meditation.

This started to feed a negative core belief about motherhood that sounded like: *"Motherhood has sucked me dry and my children are in the way of me enjoying my life."* Sure, I was ashamed to admit that I held this mindset. And yes, I knew it created more challenges and emotions of resentment and anger. Yet, I thought that if only I had more time for me—to focus on what I loved, which at the time was birth and midwifery—I would be happier. This was not the case.

I was running away from motherhood because I felt overwhelmed by the enormous responsibility, challenged by the daily mundane, and did not embody the meaning of motherhood. I had not found the joy in motherhood that we read about or sometimes experience with our friends. **I thought embracing mindfulness and practicing meditation daily would cure this discomfort.** I thought that I needed to get away from mothering in order to experience more happiness. I believed my purpose was 'out there', outside of me and separate from what was in front of me: my children. I thought I was alone and that it was all in my head—and all my fault. It didn't occur to me at the time that this was a complex problem experienced by many mothers.

And then, one day, a year after the birth of my third child, I experienced an epiphany.

My big wake-up moment was when I was about to leave my family to follow a Shaman into the Amazon to work with plant medicines so I too could become a Shaman. In my mind, I likened it to the path of Jesus or The Buddha, both spiritual masters who isolated themselves to become awakened. And awakening was the answer that I sought to get out of my misery. I remembered feeling so conflicted by this choice (and so was my husband at the time) because I was surprised that my pull to walk away from my family was so strong.

I was a stay-at-home mother who was homeschooling her children and studying and apprenticing with midwifery. And I was about to turn my back to it all, to follow a masculine-dominated way of awakening.

Thank fuckin' god, something spoke loud within.

That something is the voice of knowing, the feminine voice. And she said with conviction, *"Your work is right here, with your children, in the mundane. Not out there, not spiritually bypassing all your suffering."* I listened. And from this place forward I started to cultivate my own feminine practice of being a mindful mother and woman. And it didn't look like your typical sitting meditation practice or journeying with plant medicine, or vision-questing by fasting.

I realized that the work of motherhood is the spiritual path I am supposed to walk, not run away from. I realized that I needed to lean in more closely and, dare I use the word, *surrender* to the work of motherhood. I needed to find meaning in motherhood that gave rise to purpose. It is a path that has been gritty, hard, in my face, and real.

We use the word *authentic* all the time nowadays, and my path of motherhood gave rise to embodied authenticity. I have been truly humbled by this journey thus far, and I am only 18 years in. What follows are a few suggestions that I have learned along that way that will help to give rise to a different way of practicing mindfulness as a mother.

How to Cultivate a Practice of Mindfulness as a Modern Mother

- ★ **Begin by listening.** Listen deeply to what your interior self is saying. Practicing listening to what others say and notice what your interior says. Listen in solitude and during the chaos. Just start to listen.
- ★ **Pay attention.** Notice your thoughts, feelings, physical sensations, images and memories. Every moment we are given information about ourselves and the experience of others. We need to pay close attention to what is arising within. This can be done while cooking, nursing, playing, driving, dressing, showering, dancing, walking, shopping. Just pay attention.
- ★ **Open in love.** Blow open the cage that shields the heart and really love your children, even in their challenges. This grows love for you. This means taking risks with feelings and it usually involves tears. Commit to love.

- ★ **Stop believing your thoughts.** Find a tool or therapist that can help you challenge your thoughts and limiting beliefs. When you start to pay attention, you begin to notice the thoughts that you are believing as truth, and how those thoughts are causing you pain. When you believe your stressful thoughts, which never go away, you feel miserable. Begin a practice of inquiry.
- ★ **Be curious.** Curiosity is a beautiful friend. Lead with curiosity, rather than reason or righteousness. Be curious about your experiences and those around you.
- ★ **Find meaning in motherhood.** This is a personal quest that will look unique for every mother. Without meaning in motherhood, motherhood is one-dimensional. Meaning gives rise to purpose, and purpose gives rise to deep satisfaction (aka happiness).

The art of mindfulness can be discovered within the energy of motherhood. From my lived experience, it does not necessarily need the sitting practice of meditation. I am inviting modern mothers to contemplate this idea and to listen, really listen, and determine for yourself if these suggestions ring true. If anything, it is offering a way of being with mothering and mindfulness that is manageable and meaningful.

Bottom line: you are enough; you are doing enough.

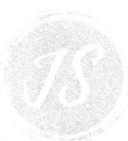

THERAPEUTIC ACTIVITY
EMBRACING YOURSELF AS A LOVING MOTHER

"What is the definition of Mothering?
Raising your child/ren to become themselves. Helping them find the balance between independence and a dependable bond. To figure out who we are and who we want to be outside of our family bonds." ~ Eliza Reynolds

After your birth experience, you may have felt disconnected from yourself, confused about your role as a mother, and possibly distant from your spouse or partner. Perhaps, something feels like it was missing and perhaps you have made note about wanting '*it*' back.

What is the '*it*' that you want to experience or regain?

Are you ready to reclaim what was lost? Only you hold the power to claim your role as a Mother and what that means for you. **You get to define this for yourself and your family.** Yourself as a Mother may have felt blurry or confusing. Not the experience you had hoped for or imagined. And this may have been a result of your childbirth experience, or perhaps your family upbringing.

You may have had good role models growing up, or you may have lacked healthy parenting role models. This module will hopefully help you reconnect to that place of knowing inside that will help to guide your way as a Mother.

In the following exercise, you are encouraged to begin re-scripting your definition of what it means to be a loving mother. Let your creative visioning juices flow.

What are the qualities and/or characteristics of a loving mother?

How does a loving mother behave?

Is a loving mother allowed to make mistakes? How would she handle her mistakes?

What are some of her 'non-negotiables'? What won't she tolerate?

What commitments is she willing to make to step powerfully into her role as a mother? From here on, what does she commit to?

Narrative Exercise

You are invited to write a letter, from your future ideal mother-self, to remind you how amazing you are as a mother. There will be times when you will doubt this about yourself, so you are writing to remember always how brave, strong, beautiful, loving, and caring you are as a mother, and how much you love your child(ren), your family, and yourself.

Dear Brave Mother, I am writing to remind you that you are…

CHAPTER 11

Reclaiming Your Birth Story

*"How you tell your story is an indicator
of how much you have healed." ~ Dan Siegel*

You have worked hard throughout this program to shift any unwanted negative feelings and thoughts pertaining to your childbirth experience. You have felt your feelings, named your pain, faced your fears, and spoke with utmost honesty.

Dr. Dan Siegel states that we can measure growth and healing, and integration from painful past events, by **how we tell our story.** The goal is to be able to share your experience in a coherent and calm way, that makes sense to you, and becomes part of the tapestry of your life's journey.

There will always be painful aspects to the telling of the story, but the shifts occur when you can share it with honest truth and hearts wide open. So, **you get to choose what you want to share, why you want to share it, and with whom.** It is your story, your experience, and your journey of healing.

Nobody else can own it, claim it, or share it.

Post traumatic growth informs us that adverse experiences cultivate grit, growth, and resilience. Life continues to present us with adverse experiences, we cannot avoid challenges and hardships. **We can, however, control how we respond to those experiences—during and afterwards.** Is it possible that your adverse childbirth experience becomes a catalyst for growth and greater resilience?

Can there be a gift hidden in the pain?

On Vulnerability

*"The truth is: Belonging starts with self-acceptance.
Your level of belonging, in fact, can never be greater than your level of self-acceptance, because believing that you're enough is what gives you the courage to be authentic, vulnerable and imperfect." ~ Brené Brown*

Vulnerability feels like your soul is exposed, turned inside out, waiting for a response. To be vulnerable requires authentically showing up in your life. It is not vulnerable to merely show up for yourself in the silence of your home. It involves relating to others or exposing a part of yourself, your soul, to another. It is the act of feeling exposed, raw, real, and open as a way of connecting that can feel like the scariest thing anyone could ever do.

Vulnerability does not feel safe, simply put.

It doesn't feel safe because, for the most part, it has not been safe to be authentic and exposed. In moments of vulnerability, we may have experienced an attack, bullying, mockery, belittling, laughter, emptiness, and more profound yet, public or family shunning. It is as if our cells recoil at the thought of being vulnerable, we move away from it. And again, we are told that we need to lean into the discomfort of vulnerability and offer more, not less, of ourselves. The world needs this, and we need this. Why do we need this?

Author Brené Brown, deemed the expert on vulnerability, suggests that human vulnerability opens our hearts and, thus, shines a light on our shame, so we no longer live small. We need to come out of our hiding places so that we can belong—genuinely belong. When we are vulnerable, we are real. And when we are real—hiding nothing and letting our imperfections be seen—we are tapping into vulnerability.

That said, vulnerability has not always been perceived as powerful. For example, I invite you to pay attention to any judgmental thoughts, felt sensations in your body, feeling reactions when you hear the phrase: *She was so vulnerable.*

What did you notice? Maybe you noticed an open reaction, curious to hear more. Or perhaps you felt constriction, fear, protection; akin to feeling 'sorry' for someone who was vulnerable. Maybe you felt anger. Or, perhaps you interpreted the phrase as an indication of weakness. As you can see, there are many possible reactions to the words: *She was so vulnerable.*

I recognize that within myself I have an array of responses depending on the context in which the statement is used. Are we referring to a woman who was writing a personal story? Or a child who was exposed to an environmental catastrophe? A teenager who was attacked while walking home from school? An executive director speaking publicly about a cause? Or, a mother in labour?

Each scenario generates a different emotional response. And yet, we praise vulnerability. From my vantage point, **vulnerability is being both powerful and powerlessness.**

It is a paradox: *to be courageous and weak.* Take into consideration the vagina—powerful, erotic, beautiful, feminine and an intimate part of a woman that can also be easily wounded, shut down, disgraced, disowned and shamed. Exposing the fragile, soft parts that can be both the gateway to joy and deep pain. The act of vulnerability is intensely feminine.

Exposing our soul in a courageously authentic way, with flaws on the outside, can produce both joy and sorrow. It is risky. Therefore, it is understandable why we are shy to show up with vulnerability in our day-to-day lives if we are still figuring out whether being vulnerable means demonstrating strength or exposing our weakness. And I would add it is extra challenging for anyone who is not of the dominant culture (that being white men who align with patriarchal values).

Jumping forward, I want to turn your attention towards the notion that when a woman is in labour and giving birth, she is utterly vulnerable. Notice what arose within you. What were your thoughts, emotions, felt sensations? Take a moment to listen to what is emerging within, what story is showing up.

Just the other day I was having a passionate conversation with some colleagues and women friends. I was speaking about how vulnerable and exposed I was feeling since sharing my first draft of my opening chapter in this guidebook. In the section, I unpacked my birth story, my shame, and my unannounced birth trauma. It was the very first time I chose to be this public about my birth experience. Part of it was cathartic, but another part was my soul's need to weave this story into my life's work so that I can show up more authentic with each mother I serve.

I was spinning out my anxiety that presented because a part of me was interpreting my decision as dangerous, ridiculous, and selfish. Moreover, I felt as if I was standing on the front lines awaiting a verbal thunderstorm of opinions raining down about one of *the most* vulnerable times of my life. What had I done? Vulnerability is bullshit, I thought to myself.

As the tension in the room was rising, we were all feeding off this angst. My colleague caught me off-guard and posed a statement: Jen, women in labour are vulnerable, period. You were incredibly vulnerable during your birth experience. And so how can you expect a woman in labour to stand up for herself, defend herself, push against unwanted procedures and protocols, or *not* hand her power over to her caregiver?

Whoa! This comment hit me on so many levels, my system was highly activated and jumping all over the place. It was as if all of my years of experience were being sorted out in my brain and I needed to pull it all together to have a response that was short and legitimate.

I babbled my way through and felt like I was making no sense at all. Women being vulnerable in labour is such a massive topic of discussion, I said. On the one hand, women are profoundly powerful in labour and birth; and right, they are also incredibly vulnerable.

How was I interpreting this idea of vulnerability? Why was I so triggered? Part of my trigger was that I said I wish women did not hand their power over to their caregivers. But I saw my error in this statement, as we collectively unpacked the concept. Granted we only skimmed the surface.

However, these questions entered my mind:

>What is power?
>Who has power?
>Where is the power?
>How is power used?
>What is vulnerability in this context?

It is fair to say that everyone in the birthing room has their power. The mother has personal power, along with the caregiver, support people, partner, family members, etc. Each person brings with them, into the room, intrinsic power. However, in this milieu, we bump up against the tension that lies between a mother's need and desire to exert her power during labour and birth, and the needs of the 'expert' in the room.

I imagine that you can already sense the complexity involved in this statement. And how appropriate it would be to do a power analysis to ascertain who holds more power in the birthing environment. That said, I am not going to unpack a power analysis here. But let's just say that those who work within and for the medical establishment hold an incredible amount of power to influence, control, inform and manage the experience of labour and birth. And fundamentally, a woman's labouring body houses a shitload of knowledge and power. Thus, one type is external power or power over, and the other is, internal power or power within.

Now, let's take into consideration that women are still victims of oppression and marginalized women, which includes women of colour, Indigenous women, Islamic women, and refugee women, experience a much higher degree of social abuse and mistreatment of care.

A patriarchal worldview foundationally informs the medical establishment. Thus, when you combine oppressed women within a patriarchal institution, you encounter power over tactics that are intended to control, manage, suppress, disempower and submit. We cannot ignore the fact that for centuries women have been raised within the dominant cultural worldview. One imprint in particular haunts women in labour: the caregiver knows best. Within this mindset, there is a power exchange that occurs, albeit invisible, and thus the caregiver inevitably has power over the labouring mother.

Does this not elicit vulnerability? The kind of vulnerability that denotes weakness and a risk of harm.

The notion above refers to the quality of vulnerability that I have been defending against for the past seventeen years. To say that a woman in labour is vulnerable is akin to saying she is in harm's way. Moreover, I am ignited to do something about this concern, and I react with a desire to protect. My backlash attempt was to empower women through education, inspiring mothers to take back their births, body, and baby. All of which was motivated by the concept: *do not allow yourself to be vulnerable in labour and delivery.*

Most of the research I explored on the topic of childbirth trauma noted that women felt disempowered and traumatized in labour when they lacked choice and control, felt violated, abandoned, neglected, or feared that there was an emergency that could have resulted in the death of their baby. To mitigate this from happening, it seemed evident at the time that we need women to feel prepared, confident, knowledgeable, trusting, and determined to be 'self-directed' in childbirth. In other words, to mitigate vulnerability (because that meant you were in harm's way) you needed inner strength, knowledge, and determination.

Thus, to be genuinely vulnerable in labour and birth was/is risky. And yet, the truth is, childbirth is entirely a journey of vulnerability and letting go. So we stand at this crossroads again. *If it is not safe to be vulnerable, because when we are vulnerable we get hurt, how is a mother going to allow her labour to open while vulnerable?* What a dilemma.

This dilemma is what challenged me that night as I was impassioned with angst and confusion. How do I address this complicated topic? Both are true: Women in labour are incredibly vulnerable, and women in labour are full of power.

And then it hit me the next morning. Of course, I couldn't sleep that night. I felt like my ideology was butting up against my colleague's words. What was it that challenged me so much? I realized I was vulnerable. I was profoundly helpless in the postpartum with my daughter when I was utterly sick. And I was disgusted with myself for being so ill because I perceived myself as being weak. Thus, I was now in harm's way.

And harm is what occurred during that 24-hour hospital stay. My vulnerability led to a violation of my body—aggressive procedures against my will. And being immobilized for two weeks, oozing mucous out of my ass, was not only humiliating, it was vulnerable.

I was terrified of being that vulnerable.

The concept of vulnerability is complex to unpack, especially as it pertains to the childbirth milieu. The deeper I go into my understanding of vulnerability, I recognize that there is a difference between being vulnerable as a way to bring my authentic self to the world and being in a vulnerable (unsafe) situation that could result in harm. The childbirth continuum and experience include both possible forms of vulnerability. Thus, discernment is critical.

Although my body may react similarly to each case, both being perceived physiologically as a potential for harm, I must engage with my mindful mind to remind myself that vulnerability does not always involve damage. Albeit, it is still a risk.

The drive to be authentic—risking rejection from the tribe, family, friends—can trigger paralysis and symptoms similar to the terror of death. This degree of terror is a result of our biological, primary need to attach securely with others, in love and kindness. If we consider the above notion, to connect with love and compassion as a primary motivation, we are inclined to lean into vulnerability as a means to meaningful *connection and belonging.*

My drive towards vulnerability, authenticity, and raw exposure of my heart's story is not something I enjoy doing: it is a necessity. Without it, my experience of life would feel empty and meaningless. It is worth the risk. And that also means that, rather than shaming myself for having been vulnerable during my birth and postpartum, I can connect with this past part and hold her in love. The antidote is a compassionate connection and non-judgemental understanding.

I sat with this chapter and contemplated the paradox of vulnerability: holding both powerfulness and powerlessness. I allowed myself to venture inside to connect to my postpartum self; grief showed up as I held my dear collapsed part in the depths of her pain of vulnerability. Knowing in that moment that I could carry both powerfulness and powerlessness within myself, and that is enough.

REFLECTIVE EXERCISE
YOUR BIRTH STORY

What aspects of your birth story do you want to hang onto?

Are there any aspects of your experience that are you still struggling to understand or accept? If so, what are they?

Notice the difference between sharing from a place of empowerment versus a place of disempowerment. What are the differences?

When you get right down to it, what is stopping you from changing the way you tell your story? What is holding you back?

THERAPEUTIC ACTIVITY
NARRATIVE EXERCISE

Take a moment and feel into **the new story you want to tell**, see yourself sharing about your birth experience and notice any felt sensations that arise. Allow yourself to fully consider this possibility of claiming a new birth story. Rich within your story is meaning, brought to the forefront by how you have made sense out of your experience. When you are ready, begin to write your new birth story. When you are done, **re-read it to yourself and try to pull out the 'meaning' in the story.** Sometimes it helps to imagine telling your birth story to your child at 1, 7, 13, 21 years of age.

The birth story I want to tell is...

After you finish writing the birth story you want to tell, take a moment to check in with yourself and ask these questions:

Where am I on my journey, how big is the gap between the story I want to tell and the story I am telling?

How close am I to telling this new story?

What is preventing me from claiming this new story?

Often, we hang onto our stories because we are afraid that if we let aspects of it go, we are letting go of the entire experience. Sometimes we cling to parts of the story in hopes that we can hold another accountable. When we step outside of the need to hang onto all the painful details of the past experience, we allow space for integration, coherence and wisdom to form. As often stated by Joe Dispenza:

> Wisdom is the end product of
> the distillation of energy and information
> that we were holding from our past adversities.

What am I still telling myself about my past childbirth experience?

What am I telling myself about myself as it pertains to this experience?

Has it changed? If yes, how? If no, why not?

If you are hearing a narrative that still sounds judging, punishing, or stressful, take a moment and write down all your stressful thoughts.

Pause.

And ask yourself, again, what do I *need* in order to liberate myself from this stressful narrative?

>   Do I need to be heard?
>   Do I need to be validated?
>   Do I need to write a letter?
>   Do I need to go to a human rights lawyer?
>   Do I need to speak about it more?
>   Do I need to cry?
>   Do I need to be witnessed?
>   Do I need to be held or touched?
>   What do you need?

There are so many different therapeutic and healing modalities that you can access to further your healing journey. This guidebook has hopefully inspired a desire to deepen your healing process and serve as a stepping stone along the way. Throughout the journey towards healing and wholeness, we stumble upon different teachers, therapists, and healers who can bless us with their wisdom and gifts.

At this stage, I invite you to consider next steps.

>   Who will you contact?
>   What would feel right for you?
>   What kind of healing modality are you drawn to?
>   What kind of support group do you want to join?

As you consider these questions, a bigger question to contemplate:

> Who will you be and who do you want to become
> at the end of this journey?

I leave you with these final thoughts...

We are informed by the past until we become conscious of it. Once we are conscious of how our past has informed how we think, feel and behave, then, and only then, can we have the power to step into a new way of being and perceiving.

If you want to perceive your childbirth through a different lens and tell your story that is authentic, real and free from trauma, then it begins with a belief that this is possible.

You will know you are liberated from the experience when you tell the story and you are no longer activated by it. And, you can see the gifts that the experience brought you, and you have integrated all the pieces. You feel whole, intact, and coherent.

We know we have healed when we tell a story that is coherent and fluid, and we can tolerate the emotional material that arises within. **You may always shed a tear when you tell your story—that is authentic.** However, the thoughts you attach to those tears will either liberate you or generate suffering.

Grief is inevitable; suffering is optional.

It is with great hope that as you worked through the content and exercises throughout this guidebook that you discovered something about yourself that you did not know existed; that you were inspired; that you received insight; and that you feel compelled to courageous step forward and heal.

When we feel, we begin to heal.

What we need in order to support healing is akin to what women need in labour and birth: *presence, security, love, kindness, choice, and belief.*

My deep heartfelt intention for all mothers who have experienced a difficult and/or traumatic childbirth is...

May the challenges you faced during your birth experience ignite the fire within your being. May you discover the profound healer within that blows open your heart with an overflowing capacity to love your family, your community, the world, and yourself with grace and ease.

One Day I Will Rage
(for my daughter)

One day I will rage.

One day I will grieve a wild prayer for humanity.

I feel it brewing within my soul,

I see the fangs snarled and dripping with blood.

One day I will scream.

Scream for all those who have been raped,

For those who have been murdered,

For those frozen in violence,

For the destruction of our earth,

For the terror our children feel,

For every mother who has suffered a devastating loss,

For every person who dies alone,

For those who have never been loved.

One day I will bare my soul.

And join the silent raging and grieving voices of humanity.

Will you join me?

Jennifer Summerfeldt

References

Badenoch, Bonnie. Being a Brain Wise Therapist: A Practical Guide to Interpersonal Neurobiology. New York, New York: W.W. Norton & Norton, 2008.

Buckley, Sarah J. "Hormonal Physiology of Childbearing: Evidence and Implications for Women, Babies, and Maternity Care." Childbirth Connection Programs: National Partnership for Women and Families, 2015.

Coates, Rose, Susan Ayers, and Richard de Visser. "Women's Experiences of Postnatal Distress: A Qualitative Study." BMC Pregnancy and Childbirth 14 (2014): 359. doi:10.1186/1471-2393-14-359.

Congdon, Jayme L., Nancy E. Adler, Elissa S. Epel, Barbara A. Laraia, and Nicole R. Bush. "A Prospective Investigation of Prenatal Mood and Childbirth Perceptions in an Ethnically Diverse, Low-Income Sample." Birth 43, no. 2 (2016). doi:10.1111/birt.12221.

Dekker, Rebecca. "Induction for Going Past Your Due Date: What Does the Evidence Say ?," 2015.

Dispenza, Joe. Breaking the Habit of Being Yourself: How to Lose Your Mind and Create a New One. Carlsbad, California: Hay House Inc., 2012.

Edwards, Sarah R, Lindsey Devries, and Aleska R Hagan. "Risk Factors for Postpartum PTSD : Coercion During Labor and History of Abuse," 2014, 10–11.

Foley, Suzanne, Rosalind Crawley, Stephanie Wilkie, and Susan Ayers. "The Birth Memories and Recall Questionnaire (BirthMARQ): Development and Evaluation." BMC Pregnancy and Childbirth 14, no. 1 (2014): 1–16. doi:10.1186/1471-2393-14-211.

Geller, Shari M, and Stephen W Porges. "Therapeutic Presence: Neurophysiological Mechanisms Mediating Feeling Safe in Therapeutic Relationships." Journal of Psychotherapy Integration, 2014. doi:10.1037/a0037511.

Grekin, Rebecca, and Michael W. O'Hara. "Prevalence and Risk Factors of Postpartum Posttraumatic Stress Disorder: A Meta-Analysis." Clinical Psychology Review 34, no. 5 (2014). doi:10.1016/j.cpr.2014.05.003.

Herman, Judith. Trauma and Recovery . 2nd ed. New York: Perseus Book Group, 1997.

Herman, Judith L. "Review of Special Issue: Guidelines for Treating Dissociative Identity Disorder in Adults (3rd Revision); Rebuilding Shattered Lives: Treating Complex PTSD and Dissociative Disorders; and Understanding and Treating Dissociative Identity Disorder: A Relati." Psychoanalytic Psychology 29, no. 2 (2012): 267–69. doi:10.1037/a0027818.

James, Stella. "Women's Experiences of Symptoms of Posttraumatic Stress Disorder (PTSD) after Traumatic Childbirth: A Review and Critical Appraisal." Archives of Women's Mental Health, 2015, 761–71. doi:10.1007/s00737-015-0560-x.

Kerr, Laura. "Live Within Your Window of Tolerance." San Fransico, CA, 2015. www.laurakerr.com

Levine, Peter A. In an Unspoken Voice: How the Body Releases Trauma and Restores Goodness. Berkeley, California: North Atlantic Books, 2010.

Main, Mary, Erik Hesse, and Siegfried Hesse. "Attachment Theory and Research: Overview with Suggested Applications to Child Custody." Family Court Review 49, no. 3 (2011): 426–63. doi:10.1111/j.1744-1617.2011.01383.x.

Mate, Gabor. "Compassionate Inquiry." Edmonton, 2017.

McGilchrist, Iain. RSA Animate: The Divided Brain. YouTube, 2011.

McKenzie-McHarg, Kirstie. "Traumatic Birth: Understanding Predictors, Triggers, and Counselling Process Is Essential to Treatment." Birth 31, no. 3 (2004): 219–21.

McKenzie-McHarg, Kirstie, Susan Ayers, Elizabeth Ford, Antje Horsch, Julie Jomeen, Alexandra Sawyer, Claire Stramrood, Gill Thomson, and Pauline Slade. "Post-Traumatic Stress Disorder Following Childbirth: An Update of Current Issues and Recommendations for Future Research." Journal of Reproductive and Infant Psychology 33, no. 3 (2015). doi:http://dx.doi.org/10.1080/02646838.2015.1031646.

Odent, M. Primal Health. London: Century Hutchinson, 1986.

Odent, Michel. The Scientification of Love. England: Free Association Books, 2000. doi:https://doi.org/10.1136/bmj.320.7245.1346.

Porges, Stephen W. "The Polyvagal Theory: New Insights into Adaptive Reactions of the Autonomic Nervous System." Cleveland Clinic Journal of Medicine, 2009. doi:10.3949/ccjm.76.s2.17.

Porges, Stephen W. "Love: An Emergent Property of the Mammalian Autonomic Nervous System." Psychoneuroendocrinology 23, no. 8 (1998): 837–61. doi:10.1016/S0306-4530(98)00057-2.

Seidmahmoodi, Jawad, Changiz Rahimi, and Norolah Mohamadi. "Resiliency and Religious Orientation: Factors Contributing to Posttraumatic Growth in Iranian Subjects." Iranian Journal of Psychiatry 6, no. 4 (2011): 145–50.

Seligman, Martin E. P., and Mihaly Csikszentmihalyi. "Positive Psychology: An Introduction." American Psychologist 55, no. 1 (2000): 5–14. doi:10.1037//0003-066X.55.1.5.

Siegel, Daniel. "The Mindful Brain: The Neurobiology of Wellbeing." 2001. doi:978-1-60407-227-3.

Siegel, Daniel J. "Toward an Interpersonal Neurobiology of the Developing Mind: Attachment Relationships, 'Mindsight,' and Neural Integration." Infant Mental Health Journal 22, no. 1–2 (2001): 67–94. doi:10.1002/1097-0355(200101/04)22:1<67::AID-IMHJ3>3.0.CO;2-G.

Siegel, Daniel J. Mindsight: The New Science of Personal Transformation. New York: Random House Publishing Group, 2010.

Siegel, Daniel J. "Practicing Mindsight." Sounds True, 2015. https://www.udemy.com/practicing-mindsight/

Simington, Jane. Trauma Recovery Certification Handbook. 6th ed. Edmonton: Taking Flight International, 2013.

WHO. "The Prevention and Elimination of Disrespect and Abuse During Facility-Based Childbirth," 2015. http://apps.who.int/iris/bitstream/10665/134588/1/WHO_RHR_14.23_eng.pdf?ua=1&ua=1

Williamson, John B., Eric C. Porges, Damon G. Lamb, and Stephen W. Porges. "Maladaptive Autonomic Regulation in PTSD Accelerates Physiological Aging." Frontiers in Psychology 5, no. January (2015): 1–12. doi:10.3389/fpsyg.2014.01571.

ABOUT THE AUTHOR

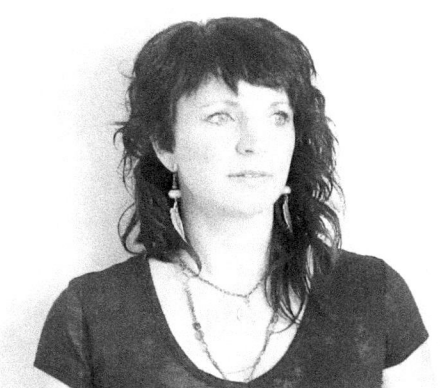

Jennifer Summerfeldt holds an MA in Counselling Psychology and has nearly two decades of experience in maternal health and psychology. In addition to being a counsellor and a coach, Jennifer has also been a childbirth advocate, maternal educator, doula, midwifery apprentice, and published writer. She uses her expertise and voice to help advance the dialogue on motherhood, mental health, and healing. To contact Jennifer for speaking events or apply for her program, visit www.jennifersummerfeldt.com

www.ingramcontent.com/pod-product-compliance
Lightning Source LLC
Chambersburg PA
CBHW081445070526
44586CB00019B/2235